Dr Peta Wright is a gynaecologist and fertility specialist. She completed her undergraduate medical degree with Honours at Monash University and obtained her RANZCOG Fellowship in 2013. She has completed a Masters of Reproductive Medicine and a certificate in Women's Integrative Medicine. Peta is deeply committed to all aspects of women's healthcare and founded Vera Women's Wellness in 2021. She strives to take a holistic approach to optimising the health of women of all ages. It is Peta's purpose in life to help women remember the magic and beauty in their bodies and help to create a society that honours women and supports them to feel safe in their bodies and in the world.

HEALING PELVIC PAIN

Dr Peta Wright

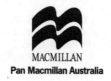

MACMILLAN
Pan Macmillan Australia

Pan Macmillan acknowledges the Traditional Custodians of Country throughout Australia and their connections to lands, waters and communities. We pay our respect to Elders past and present and extend that respect to all Aboriginal and Torres Strait Islander peoples today. We honour more than sixty thousand years of storytelling, art and culture.

First published 2023 in Macmillan by Pan Macmillan Australia Pty Ltd
1 Market Street, Sydney, New South Wales, Australia, 2000

A catalogue record for this book is available from the National Library of Australia

Typeset in 11/15.5 pt Sabon LT Std by Midland Typesetters, Australia

Printed by IVE

Lyrics on pages 252–3 from 'Your Blood Is Amazing' reproduced with kind permission from Lucy Peach.

Case histories included in this book are de-identified and fictionalised compilations of representative cases for the purposes of illustration only. Any resemblance to persons living or dead is purely coincidental.

The author and the publisher have made every effort to contact copyright holders for material used in this book. Any person or organisation that may have been overlooked should contact the publisher.

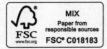

The paper in this book is FSC® certified. FSC® promotes environmentally responsible, socially beneficial and economically viable management of the world's forests.

This book was written on Jinibara Country.

For all my patients, who are the reason I do this work.
Your stories have taught me more than I could ever learn
at medical school, and you inspire me every day. May you
all know the magic and wisdom of your body.

Contents

'Even if our minds forget. Every memory, pleasant or painful, has a nervous system signature. Our memories live in the body as sensation. No matter who caused the sensation, it is ours to free when we're ready. Inhale. Exhale. Welcome to presence.' – Liz Letchford

HEALING PELVIC PAIN

Introduction:
In search of true healing

The meaning of *heal* is to make free from injury or disease: to make sound or whole.

Healing is a word we rarely hear in modern medicine – outside the description of 'a healing wound'. It is certainly rarely used to describe the way doctors work with patients. Healing is thought of as something energy workers, shamans or, dare I say it, witches might claim to do.

Pelvic pain affects one in five women and, in my experience as a gynaecologist, appears to be a growing problem despite the increasing awareness and attention it has garnered recently from the medical profession, government and community at large. I think the problem we face when we think about pelvic pain and endometriosis is best described in the slight difference between the two halves of the accepted definition of healing above. The biomedical model used by modern medicine concentrates on the first – to make free from injury or disease – by seeking a single structural cause for disease and aiming to rid the body of it.

As a women's health practitioner and advocate, and based on the currently available literature, I believe this is failing women and breaking doctors' Hippocratic oath by doing more harm than good.

Recently the Australian government announced an inquiry into misogyny in medicine, but even the politicians and the journalists leading the campaign were describing misogyny as too few women being offered or having access to surgery for chronic pelvic pain. Many women and those in power think that the answer to women's pain is validating it by doing an operation. Operations are expensive, but a hell of a lot less expensive and far more simple than the system-wide change and fresh approach I believe we need.

The current approach to pelvic pain is at odds with the second part of the definition of 'heal' – to make whole. This is my definition of healing, and mapping out a pathway to true healing for women with pelvic pain is my aim in this book. From where I'm sitting, after 17 years of working with women experiencing pain and being trained within the current medical system, I know what's not working and what does work for the women who come to see me.

> While I use the terms women and girls throughout this book for simplicity – I mean it to include people assigned female at birth or who have any variation of female anatomy. I treat many people who identify as non-binary or transgender but who may also experience things like pelvic pain, periods and ovulation.

I believe that as a society we make men the standard, while women – and all the ways we deviate from that linear masculinity through our menstrual cycle, which is by definition nonlinear – are treated as 'abnormal' or 'pathological' (diseased). If women can't behave the same way every day of their cycle, be productive every day of their cycle, then the medical instinct is to conclude their bodies are defective and must be diagnosed.

I totally reject this paradigm of pathologisation that plagues most 'conditions' in gynaecology. More often than not, the suffering that women experience comes from a lack of education (among doctors and patients alike) about what's normal; the pressure to conform or fit into a society that makes it difficult to nurture a female body; the normal physiological response of the body to its environment; the detrimental effects of a dangerous environment on a woman's body; or significant trauma. In most cases it's the society that's pathological, not the woman's body.

My idea of true healing is not just helping to heal the body and pelvic pain in a vacuum. If we continue to focus on trying to heal a woman without considering her environment and the way her nervous system, immune system and hormonal system change in response to that environment, we will continue to miss the point.

I know that when working with a woman and treating her as a whole, considering the mind–body–environment continuum is effective. This approach doesn't view a woman as diseased or broken but just disconnected from herself. It's about reminding her of the wholeness that's there inside her and has always been. True healing comes by empowering women and reminding them of how amazing their bodies really are. When women are comfortable in their full power, that will be the paradigm shift we have been waiting for.

As I began to see more and more women through this more holistic lens, I realised that time, care and love were just as important as drugs, surgery and physiotherapy or any other standard treatments – if not more so. This is, in essence, the first part of establishing safety and stability for the traumatised nervous system – which nearly every patient with chronic pain has. Providing a safe, grounded presence so that the patient simply feels cared for is termed co-regulation. It was never taught to me at medical school, but it's the single most important aspect of healing chronic pain. As I began to understand co-regulation and all the other things that help create a deeper sense of nervous-system safety, I started to dream of a different model of care – one that aimed from the very first visit to instil a sense of safety, stability and bodily autonomy in the women who came to see me.

That dream turned into a holistic women's health centre grounded in nature.

In 2020, in the midst of the Covid-19 pandemic, I came to the realisation that I was part of the problem. I had been seeing woman after woman, every day from 6 am to 6 pm, who told me the same stories – chronic pain, severe premenstrual symptoms and chronic stress. I became burnt out too. I was giving advice about the importance of exercise, sleep and taking time for self-care, but I wasn't taking my own advice. I realised that if I wanted my message to have real power, I needed to start with myself and take the time to live more cyclically. I also realised that getting to the root of complex problems such as chronic pelvic pain takes time and energy, and if I wanted to give women the best care I could, I needed to ensure that I had enough time to recharge.

These realisations were the beginning of Vera Women's Wellness – a space for holistic care that seeks to educate and empower women, and work with them to get to the often deep roots of their health issues. Nestled in the foothills near the Brisbane CBD, it forces women to take time out for themselves and showcases the power of nature in healing.

At the practice, we celebrate and support the female body, and each person who comes is reminded that they are in charge of their body and already hold great wisdom about it and what's right for them. Our job as practitioners is mostly guiding women back to themselves and supporting them to make changes that nourish and nurture their bodies rather than diagnosing disease and dysfunction. A very real part of the healing that happens here is the building of a community. In this book, I have drawn extensively from my experience of working with women in this way, and I want to provide you with the same approach to healing pelvic pain you might find at Vera.

As a practitioner, I see many women with chronic pelvic pain, often after as many as eight surgeries have left them in as much or more pain than before their first. I see women who are looking for the fix to their chronic pain only in their pelvis, when I know this is only going to address part of the problem. True healing can never be found only by looking in the pelvis with a camera – which is why it so often fails. We need to dig deeper, layer by layer through what, at surface level, seems like the whole problem (endometriosis) down into the roots of pain and suffering.

The holistic framework I use as a practitioner for healing pelvic pain encompasses helping women learn about their body, reduce their fear, nurture themselves, calm their nervous system, map their pain story, rewire their nervous system, reduce tension in their body, celebrate their body, and find a way to true healing so that they can live their life on their own terms.

This is what this book will teach you – providing you with the tools you need to get to the roots of your pain, become empowered and free yourself from suffering.

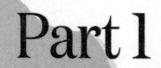

Part 1

What causes pelvic pain?

1

Periods and pelvic pain

Your body is a masterpiece. Before we examine the origins and consequences of pelvic pain, we will start in the place we've neglected for too long – a place to celebrate the wonder of our body, our hormones and our menstrual cycle, of everything that makes us awe-inspiring and magical. Don't skip this section if you're a woman who experiences pain. Don't think this doesn't apply to you. Don't think there's no beauty for you to see. It applies to you even more.

Demystifying our menstrual cycle

Too often in Western culture, the period is seen as unnatural or at the very least inconvenient. But it's a part of who we are, and the first step towards healing is knowing the way things should be. Understanding our menstrual cycle is the foundation for understanding how our environment and lifestyle can impact the health of our hormones, and the way our biology changes as we flow across the cycle.

A normal cycle

The menstrual cycle ends and begins with your period, and day 1 of the cycle is the first day of bleeding. Many guides will break down the menstrual cycle into only two phases – follicular (pre-ovulation) and luteal (post-ovulation) – but there are four distinct hormonal phases that mirror the seasons of the natural world:

Week 1: Menstrual phase – winter

Week 2: Follicular phase – spring

Week 3: Ovulatory/early luteal phase – summer

Week 4: Late luteal phase – autumn.

Our hormones and menstrual cycle are under the control of a gland in the brain called the hypothalamus. She is like the CEO, with another gland called the pituitary gland her second-in-command. This powerhouse duo controls not only our sex hormones (oestrogen, progesterone and testosterone), but also our thyroid (the gland in the neck that controls metabolism and growth), and our metabolic and stress hormones. Hormones are chemical messengers that get things done in the body.

The hormones involved

Because hormones are so crucial to how our bodies feel and operate daily, it's important to understand their role in this incredible hormonal symphony that takes place in our body.

Brain hormones

- **FSH:** follicle stimulating hormone, made in the pituitary gland, tells the ovaries to start maturing a developing follicle in the ovary that contains an egg.
- **LH:** luteinising hormone, made in the pituitary gland, causes ovulation when there is a mature dominant follicle in the ovary.

Ovarian hormones

- **Oestrogen:** made in the ovaries by the growing follicle, promotes growth of the endometrial lining of the uterus (in case a fertilised egg is implanted there with pregnancy). Oestrogen also promotes plump and healthy collagen and skin, and fat distribution in the breasts and hips. It boosts the brain by increasing serotonin, dopamine and oxytocin levels, making us feel happier, more productive and energetic, and it helps with memory and building our brain.

Oestrogen is muscle-building, and is crucial for strong bones. It also helps with insulin sensitivity and metabolism.

- **Testosterone:** made in the ovaries and the adrenal glands, helps support strong muscles, and increases stamina, energy and libido. It also helps build confidence and encourages risk-taking.
- **Progesterone:** made in the ovaries *only* after ovulation, supports implantation of an embryo by helping the endometrial lining of the uterus become receptive. It increases our metabolic rate and helps us relax and chill out, combating anxiety and helping with sleep. By keeping testosterone in check, it makes our hair shiny and our skin glow, and helps prevent acne. It prevents our periods being too heavy by balancing the effects of oestrogen on the lining of the uterus. It even offers anti-inflammatory and immune system support.

The hypothalamus takes in information from the environment and the rest of our body about whether it's 'safe' to kick off the menstrual cycle. As you're about to learn, making hormones and growing and releasing an egg (let alone growing and birthing a baby) are major events that require a lot of energy, so our hypothalamus won't get things going if it senses danger or lack in our environment.

The hypothalamus is affected by hormones such as insulin, thyroid hormones, leptin and ghrelin (hormones involved in metabolism), as well as cortisol and melatonin (our stress and sleep hormones respectively). If we're undereating or overexercising, or are emotionally or physically stressed, our clever hypothalamus protects us by suppressing the hormones that start the menstrual cycle in the first place, because it knows a pregnancy could put far too much stress on a body that's in danger.

However, if everything is balanced in your body and your brain has given hormone-making the go-ahead this month, the start of your cycle will find us at week 1 with menstruation.

The stages of your menstrual cycle

Week 1: days 1–7
The lining of the uterus (the uterine lining or the endometrium) has shed due to falling oestrogen and progesterone levels, as the egg you released in the previous cycle was not fertilised. For most women bleeding lasts between three and seven days. **Your hormone levels are at their lowest point in the cycle and the endometrium becomes bare – like a tree during winter preparing for a new season of growth to begin.** Mild pain or discomfort in the few days before and first few days of your period can be a normal reflection of the inflammatory process of the uterus lining shedding as studies show up to 93 per cent of girls and women report some pain with periods. Pain and discomfort are usually the result of the uterus contracting and the release of inflammatory chemicals called prostaglandins, which are released as the lining prepares to come away. It is important to understand that most women report some period pain so some level of pain is normal due to the inflammation that needs to occur for a period to happen.

Week 2: days 7–13
The low ovarian hormone levels at menstruation trigger the brain to start sending FSH down to the ovaries. FSH then stimulates the ovaries to start growing a follicle that contains a mature egg. As the follicle grows it makes oestrogen. While oestrogen affects almost every system in our body, in terms of the menstrual cycle it prompts the uterus to grow a beautiful thick lining like a little nest for an embryo to implant into.

The ovary also makes a little testosterone just before ovulation, which helps libido during this phase. Oestrogen rises, reaching a peak just before ovulation when the egg is mature. This phase sees growth in spades! **The ovarian follicle is blossoming, oestrogen and testosterone are reaching skyward, and the uterine lining is blooming into a thick, fertile carpet – this phase reflects spring.**

Week 3: days 14–21

The ovary uses oestrogen to communicate back to the brain that there's a ripe juicy egg ready to be released, triggering the brain to send back a second message in the form of LH. The LH helps the egg with its final maturation and kicks off ovulation – the release of the egg from the follicle and out into the fallopian tube, where it begins its journey in the hope of meeting up with a lucky sperm.

If fertilisation occurs, it usually takes place in the 12–24 hours after ovulation after which time the egg with wither and die. The ability to get pregnant around this time does extend to around five days, because this is the length of time sperm can live inside a woman if sex has occurred in the preceding few days. But this is the window – around five days out of a 28–30-day cycle. Contrary to what we are often led to believe, women are not fertile the whole month long.

Around ovulation, you may experience some pain due to the release of prostaglandins, which also help facilitate the release of the egg. Some of the fluid around the follicle spills into the pelvis and may also stimulate pain receptors. If you do experience some mild pain or discomfort, this means your ovaries are working just as they should.

Managing stress, reducing inflammatory foods, and taking supplements and medications that reduce inflammation (see Chapter 10) can help lessen any distressing pain at this time.

Because the follicle that the egg came from was making the oestrogen and it burst, oestrogen takes a little dip just after ovulation. The old follicle becomes the corpus luteum (Latin for 'yellow body').

The corpus luteum, an amazing hormone-producing powerhouse, continues to make oestrogen, which rises again just after ovulation to support the uterine lining. It also produces our other major reproductive hormone, progesterone.

Progesterone is crucial for implantation, as it prepares the uterine lining to become receptive to the embryo and help it nestle in. **Progesterone and oestrogen are both high during this phase, reflecting the abundance of summer.**

When the egg isn't fertilised, the corpus luteum starts to fade.

(If the egg is fertilised, the tiny embryo will continue to make its way into the uterus and implant in the nest of the uterine lining. The placenta and baby will grow, causing oestrogen and progesterone to skyrocket for the next nine months, and you won't get your period because both of these hormones support the growth of that endometrial lining to keep it strong and stable.)

Week 4: days 22-28

As the corpus luteum shrinks further, oestrogen and progesterone start to drop in the week before your period.

Because the endometrial lining is dependent upon both oestrogen and progesterone to sustain a strong and stable nest, as the hormone levels plummet the endometrium gets ready to shed. **The shedding of the lining and falling away of hormones are just like autumn leaves falling from a tree.**

As the endometrial cells start to break down, they also make prostaglandins, which may set off uterine cramping and ultimately the arrival of your period and the return of winter. The cycle is complete, and you are back to week 1.

Sometimes, particularly because of how little support girls and women are given with their cycles and periods, things don't go entirely according to this plan. This can lead to distressing pain and suffering that we will examine and look to heal in this book.

Jess's pain story, part 1

Jessica began telling me her pain story. At first it was just with her periods but now she was in pain every day. Jessica was 28 but her pain began around 14. She was prescribed the Pill by a GP, which didn't help, and she went on to have her first laparoscopy (keyhole exploratory surgery of the pelvis) at 19. The laparoscopy revealed mild endometriosis (tissue like the uterine lining found outside the uterus in the pelvis), which the surgeon ablated (burnt away). Despite this surgery, Jess's pain returned shortly after. Her initial gynaecologist didn't feel that more surgery was warranted and so Jess sought a second opinion.

Jess found a surgeon who made her feel validated and who, over the course of the next eight years, performed seven more laparoscopies to remove endometriosis. Jess reported some relief for a short period after each surgery, but her pain always returned. With each pain flare, her gynaecologist recommended another laparoscopy. At her last laparoscopy the surgeon found no significant endometriosis, but her specialist organised an ultrasound and diagnosed her with adenomyosis – a condition like endometriosis but where the endometrial cells grow in the muscular wall of the uterus instead of inside the pelvis. Her pain was now attributed to adenomyosis.

Jess was prescribed the oral contraceptive Pill, extra progestin (synthetic hormones to suppress ovulation and periods), a hormonal IUD (intrauterine device) and even a drug to switch off the ovaries and induce a temporary menopausal state. None of these solutions made a long-term difference to Jessica's pain, and many had intolerable side effects. Jess had even tried pelvic floor Botox injections and pelvic nerve blocks to relax the pelvic floor muscles, with no success.

She was referred to a pain specialist after she became dependent on opiate pain medications. She undertook intensive pain education programs to understand what was happening to her body and try to take control back. She tried all the nerve pain (neuromodulating) drugs available, which help quieten down pain signals in the body. These were also unsuccessful for Jess.

Jess had seen a naturopath and dietician and had tried low-FODMAP, anti-inflammatory and gluten-free diets, as well as a multitude of supplements. While eating more healthily helped her feel a little better, it wasn't a fix. She still had pain.

Jess's pain grew so bad that she became increasingly depressed and at times suicidal because of its effect on her quality of life. This was possibly a side effect of her hormonal medication, as was her weight gain and acne. Her gynaecologist started her on antidepressants to improve her mood, but these came with more troubling side effects.

She began seeing a psychiatrist, who tried different anti-depressants, antipsychotics and mood stabilisers, including lithium. These did not help. Side effects such as weight gain, drowsiness, agitation and sexual dysfunction were not worth any effect that the drugs may have had on her pain or mental state. And she still had pain.

Despite her persistent pain, Jess told me she had her own business that she loved, she was single and she had a very close relationship with her parents. She described her childhood as idyllic.

Jessica told me she felt totally broken. She was defeated and almost angry as she told me her story. She was in pain every day, despite all the medical interventions, and no longer trusted her body – or doctors for that matter. She identified wholly with being a sufferer of a chronic illness. In her mind she had not one but two chronic illnesses – endometriosis and adenomyosis. They are both incurable and she believed that her chances of having a baby were very slim. She was counselled that if she ever wanted a baby, she should go straight to IVF rather than to try naturally.

She didn't know what else to do or who else to see, but wanted someone to fix or take away the pain she was in. By the time she saw me at Vera Women's Wellness, she was only taking the oral contraceptive Pill. She had realised that the other drugs and any further surgeries were not sustainable and unlikely to be effective as a pain-management strategy.

When I asked Jess, after her decade of struggle with chronic illness, what she felt were the ongoing drivers of her pain, she said that she understood that her body's pain-signalling system was faulty and overactive because of her endometriosis and adenomyosis, but she was unable to soothe it.

Even though her last laparoscopy had revealed no endometriosis, she told me her uterus was 'riddled with adenomyosis' and that this was now likely the source of her pain. She felt constantly unsafe in her body, not knowing whether to trust her bodily sensations and unable to trust doctors – given her body was now in a worse state than when all her pain started as a teenager.

I wish Jess's story was rare. The shocking truth is that Jess is representative of a huge number of typical patients I have seen throughout my years as a gynaecologist. Needless to say, I did not do another surgery for Jess and in 'Jess's pain story, part 2' (page 14) you'll hear how Jess discovered the source of her pain. But first, let's look at how Jess got into this mess.

Our flawed view of pelvic pain

Does Jess's story describe the ravages of endometriosis and adenomyosis as a major cause of pelvic pain and disease among young women and people with female anatomy? Is endometriosis, an incurable disease that has been ignored while women suffered silently over the years, only now starting to attract the attention, research and awareness needed for women to be taken seriously and treated promptly? I think the answer to both questions is no.

Let's consider the facts of Jess's story, and those of many other women like her. She found a gynaecologist early on who identified endometriosis as a possible cause and acted promptly with surgical and hormonal intervention. She was not ignored. She was validated. She was taken seriously. She was treated – repeatedly – to the point that she began to believe she was at war with her own female biology and that any relief from her pain was out of her hands. She became reliant on an outside authority to 'remove endometriosis lesions' and be responsible for fixing her pain.

Jess and all the other women given these treatments are rendered so powerless that they come to believe their body is broken and continually needs fixing by something outside of them.

What this story actually illustrates is that there are missing pieces when it comes to our understanding of period pain and our approach to pelvic pain in women. As long as these missing pieces go unexplored and unnamed, the current medical paradigm will continue to place endometriosis and adenomyosis at the centre of the pain puzzle. But I believe that for many women these conditions have become the scapegoat for their very real pain.

Chasing only endometriosis means that women and doctors are singularly focused on endometriosis lesions and not the entirety of the woman in their office. As you can see from Jess's story, multiple surgeries to remove lesions are in most cases not only ineffective but often make pain worse by further sensitising pain pathways and creating scar tissue. The current approach not only misses the big drivers of pain, allowing them to go undetected and untreated, but also contributes to women's suffering by placing the 'solution' out of their hands and reinforcing the view that to be a woman is to suffer.

Our culture of period fear

For the women undergoing this kind of management, the potential harm is obvious, but the more insidious harm is for our girls and young women who are starting on their journeys through life. While we need better treatment for women like Jess who already have severe pain, we also need to begin at the beginning and think about the reasons why women develop debilitating pain in the first place.

Our girls are taught that if they have period pain, they might have endometriosis. Think about endometriosis now. Does it make you fearful? We don't quite know why we feel fear, but in recent times we've been taught that any period pain is not normal and that if you have period pain you should think of endometriosis.

We know that endometriosis is a common disease in women that can cause infertility and that there is often a big delay in diagnosis, given diagnosis requires laparoscopic surgery.

When I explore this fear with young women, they describe endometriosis as a dark shadowy monster lurking in their pelvis, spreading disease and destruction. The scariest part is that because they can't see it, their imagination conjures up the most frightening of scenes. They have an idea that if we shed light on it by looking with a laparoscopy, the unknown will become known and the fear will go away. They also have the impression that it is always progressive and that surgery can stop it spreading and becoming more severe. But as you will see, the truth is that the evidence simply doesn't support this.

It seems to me that we are almost conditioning our young girls to be afraid of their bodies and their periods. While I agree wholeheartedly that significant pain does need prompt help and treatment, I disagree with the idea that everyone with period pain needs surgery to look for endometriosis. I fear for a world where this has become the gold standard of care. I also feel that we need to balance these fears with counter-information and to celebrate the incredible intelligence of our female bodies.

Conditioning our young girls to fear their periods and the possibility of a lurking endometriosis monster is almost like the nocebo effect. The nocebo effect is the opposite of the placebo effect; it describes the situation where a negative effect occurs from a treatment due to a belief that the treatment will cause harm. If you tell someone enough times that something is going to be hard and painful, it often is. On the other hand, if we teach girls that mild pain is normal and support them by altering their environment and making it easier for them to care for their body rather than conditioning them to power on through like their brothers, regardless of their differing physiology, then we may alleviate their fear and suffering.

The millions of dollars spent on surgery for pelvic pain are failing women. While I agree that there is still much to learn, especially about rare severe endometriosis, we do know enough to understand that most of the time it is only part of the pain puzzle. While doctors' focus remains locked on endometriosis lesions, we are missing the deeper, larger, far more pervasive pieces of the puzzle, and our 'treatment' will often harm more women than it will help. At medical school I was trained only to look as far as endometriosis lesions, but years of noticing the missing pieces in women's stories have trained me to put down the surgeon's knife more often than not and listen.

> Our approach to pelvic pain needs to be truly integrative, with all the pieces identified and put together to represent the complexity and oneness of the body, mind and spirit.

So it was with Jess.

Jess's pain story, part 2

Jess said she had not suffered any trauma and that her only ongoing stress in her life was dealing with her chronic disease.

When I dug deeper, however, I learned that she had experienced verbal and physical bullying at high school. I learned that during her adolescence her well-meaning parents had placed high expectations on her to be a certain kind of person. I learned that she believed their love and acceptance were conditional on her playing a role that deep down she did not want to play.

Jess often felt she had to hide parts of herself to be accepted and loved. While at university, she entered a relationship that covertly became abusive. On the outside she was studying and on her path to a respectable career with a lovely boyfriend. The reality was that his abuse was getting worse and Jess ended up in hospital with serious injuries because of domestic violence. Although she eventually found the courage to leave her relationship, she was too afraid to tell her parents or anyone else about the abuse because she was ashamed of shattering the illusion of being the perfect daughter with the perfect life.

Around this time, Jess experienced her first major pelvic pain flare and had her first laparoscopy. Her diagnosis of endometriosis fostered a new level of compassion, love and care from her parents.

She then disclosed a sexual trauma that had occurred recently – again coinciding with a worsening of her pain. Like the domestic violence years before, Jess kept this experience secret, knowing it wasn't her fault, but holding onto a feeling of shame that she held inside her alongside the trauma and fear.

This is the story of a woman who was so disconnected from her own body and experiences that she didn't even recognise these multiple big-T traumas in her life.

By recognising these assaults on her nervous system and laying them out alongside her pain flares over time, Jessica was finally able to see the huge physical and emotional toll that living a double life and not feeling safe enough with the people she loved to be her authentic self had had on her body. Not to mention the more obvious effects of physical and sexual trauma.

It was no wonder she felt unsafe in her body when she didn't feel safe to show up as herself in any part of her life. Anything that deviated from the script of being perfect filled her with shame and was trapped like a hard knot in her body. Her parents were supportive – especially around her physical pain – which perhaps was part of the fuel, but it was her emotional pain that really needed to be seen, heard and validated.

Every treatment Jess had been offered aimed to reduce inflammation, suppress hormones and stifle pain signals, but the pain wouldn't stop. It buzzed incessantly within her, sometimes screaming to be heard. What if all it needed was to be listened to at last? What if the pain was an important messenger trying to get Jess to listen to her inner voice? By trying to shoot the messenger, perhaps the accepted treatment paradigm only makes the message louder.

What is your pain trying to tell you?

This book will help you see that your pelvic pain is not simply the result of a lesion or all in your head. We need to learn to listen and uncover the missing pieces that live in the space between mind and body. A detailed and real physiological sequence links trauma and chronic stress to pain and around again in a vicious cycle. Unless we can become aware of these pieces and learn to talk about them, they will remain unseen. This is the real issue.

It is often said that endometriosis takes seven years to diagnose from the first symptom. But the nervous system's response to chronic stress and trauma often goes undiagnosed for many more years. Failing to recognise this link contributes to ongoing pain and suffering, wreaking havoc on the rest of the body over time and leading to all the other stress-related conditions that run rife in our modern society.

Failing to recognise the effect of trauma, stress and environment on pain – for Jess and everyone like her – leaves women facing more problems than when they started, trapped in the belief that their own body is the enemy. But more often than not, their pain is their imprisoned and wounded inner child simply wanting to be seen, heard and expressed.

Many factors are of course involved in the development of complex pain, but my 17 years as a gynaecologist have led me to the truth that trauma and its downstream effects are too often overlooked and ignored in favour of surgical and medical procedures that can exacerbate the problem. This book will help you discover if trauma and chronic stress are part of your story, and if so to understand how they affect your physical body and your perception of pain. Even if your pain doesn't stem from an obvious trauma, the experience of pain is highly stressful. In a society that doesn't nurture and honour women, which treats pain as something to be constantly afraid of, this stress and fear often perpetuates the pain cycle. And medical trauma doesn't help. If trauma or stress are a feature of your story, this book will help you address all the pieces in your pain puzzle and see living in your body as a positive experience rather than seeing it as an enemy to be 'managed' into submission.

True healing from pelvic pain is possible. You just need to find all the pieces of the puzzle and have some support and help to put them together. The resulting picture should not just be you managing a chronic illness, but you living a full and meaningful life.

Chapter summary

- The normal menstrual cycle consists of four distinct phases – menstrual, follicular, ovulatory and luteal – all with different hormone levels and physiological, mood and metabolic changes.
- Ovulation and menstruation are both inflammatory events due to the release of prostaglandins.
- More than 90 per cent of women report some pain with their period.
- Suffering and extreme pain with periods may have more to do with a lack of support, knowledge and a culture of fear when it comes to women's bodies and periods.
- Focusing only on endometriosis or adenomyosis may be hurting rather than helping women and contributing to increasing fear and period pain.

2

Women and pain

Pain and suffering seem to have afflicted women since Eve. In our ancestral lineage as women, in our culture and in the stories that have seeped into our veins, we have been conditioned to expect pain.

Women in the Western world grow up fearing the pain of monthly bleeds and of childbirth. We learn that as we move from girlhood into womanhood, we leave behind shameless, unselfconscious moment-to-moment joy and inherit a collective sense of shame and embarrassment. We absorb the understanding that to live in a female body is not just to know pain but to suffer.

There is no celebration as we move from girlhood to womanhood, from motherhood to the wise-woman years. Instead we expect fear, shame, silence and suffering at each new metamorphosis of our incredible bodies. These are the stories we are told about how life is for women. No wonder we suffer.

As a gynaecologist, I hear over and over again the deep-seated belief that to be a woman is to be intrinsically broken. Many of the women and girls I see are at war with their own bodies. In their minds, our hormones, our menstrual cycles, our blood are the poison that hold us back, and our female biology is *the* cause of our suffering. When we grow up with this view of our own body, the cards are stacked against us. How can we win when to have a uterus is 'bleurgh and yucky' at best, debilitating at worst? While a new wave of women is now wanting to take back their power and rewrite the narrative, it's still an overwhelmingly gloomy and ugly place.

All this awareness should have led to better treatments and a lessening of the problem, but in the Western world we're at almost epidemic levels of pelvic pain. Worldwide, 14–32 per cent of women experience persistent pelvic pain, including more than 1 million in Australia, and one in nine women have been diagnosed with endometriosis. A recent Australian study of teenagers and young women found that up to 93 per cent of girls experience period pain each month, and about 20 per cent need to miss school or other activities during their periods. The spotlight on period pain and endometriosis has never been brighter, so why do suffering and pain continue to be an enormous problem? I would argue that pain and suffering don't need to go together, that you can have one without the other, and that the suffering is the most important thing to address.

Period and pelvic pain are the most common reason women come into my office, and I've come to believe that the current medical treatments are potentially doing more harm than good. Those women are almost always confused about what's causing their pain, but they're all aware of, and fear, endometriosis. They know that sometimes painful periods can be associated with endometriosis and that an operation is usually needed to diagnose or treat it. They're often not aware of many other factors at play that are well within their own control. They often don't know that there are other options, and that surgery has considerable limitations. Unless you're already seeing a health practitioner or team with a holistic view of pelvic pain, you too may automatically think of endometriosis whenever you think of troubling period or pelvic pain. Education is absolutely key in improving this situation for women and people with female anatomy. The lens through which information is delivered is also incredibly important. Is it fear-based or empowering?

Period and pelvic pain are not new. They've existed since the dawn of time. But the extent of suffering and the identification of women with their pain or with their endometriosis is increasing. So how did we get here? Can we follow the breadcrumbs back through the ages to learn how?

From antiquity until relatively recently, the observations of and 'discoveries' about period and pelvic pain have been largely made by men, with the occasional contribution from women themselves or from female healers. The conventional view of pain in women has therefore become one of someone on the outside looking in. Until the last hundred years or so, those in control – namely men – have largely written the story, and their script has become intertwined with our view of ourselves as women. It has become part of the story we tell ourselves about our body.

Only when we begin to identify where these thoughts and feelings have come from can we begin to question them. Our feelings of not-enough-ness and brokenness seem deep, but they've been handed down to us through the ages. Not only that, but many of the stories of women's power and knowledge have been hidden, so that thousands of years later we are still disconnected from our power.

A BRIEF HISTORY OF PERIOD AND PELVIC PAIN

Most stories about medicine begin with Hippocrates, a Greek physician who is widely regarded as the father of modern medicine and lived around 2500 years ago. He described many illnesses, including gynaecological conditions. He and his followers, including Plato and Aristotle (and many other practitioners for centuries), believed that a 'wandering uterus', especially in unwed and childless women, was responsible for any number of ills. If a woman didn't fulfil her societal obligations of marriage and motherhood, the uterus, devoid of purpose, would go wandering around the body, bumping into the liver or the spleen and causing not only pain but all manner of bodily malfunctions.

Women were seen as deformed or mutilated males, and menstrual discharge was even described as impure semen lacking a soul. Because of the observation that pain most often afflicted virgins, widows and unmarried women, the mainstay of recommendations in ancient times was marriage at 14 or 15, followed by a lifetime of childbearing, breastfeeding and raising children. This was the ancient equivalent of menstrual suppression with the Pill.

During the Middle Ages in Europe (c. 600–1500 CE), the Catholic Church largely controlled knowledge and leaned towards supernatural causes for illness, particularly demonic possession. The church forbade the pagan worship of female deities and began to demonise women, in Eve's image, as agents of the Devil. Medicine was still practised and taught, however, and the Trotulan gynaecology manual – published by an arguably female Italian physician in the 12th century – described uterine suffocation as a cause for pelvic pain.

During the Renaissance from the 16th century, suffocation of the uterus began to be referred to as hysteria, hysteric fits or dysregulated vapours (menstruation). Ambroise Paré, France's leading physician, agreed that the women most likely to be afflicted were virgins and widows, but added married women who abstained from sex.

In the 17th century, pain symptoms and hysteria were seen as a sign of demonic possession or witchcraft, and women were tried and punished or killed for causing such symptoms in other women. Psychological factors did begin to be seen as a possible cause for gynaecological symptoms, but only with the moral overlay that sinful, lascivious, attention-seeking women were the ones afflicted. In other words, women were often blamed for their own illnesses.

Although some proposed psychological–neurological theories of pain, the age of anatomy and dissection fostered the idea that every cause of pain was visible as disease in the body. A German doctor, Daniel Schrön, was perhaps the first to describe the lesions of endometriosis in 1690. He was also the first to suggest the theory of retrograde menstruation into the pelvis, and to recommend surgery as 'the principal remedy' to remove the 'ulcers'. It is possible, however, that Schrön was writing about pelvic inflammatory disease rather than endometriosis.

In the 19th century, surgery grew in popularity and success, and autopsies for medical students also began to flourish. Pathologists began to hunt more earnestly for correlations between symptoms and observations in a patient, and lesions found at autopsy. French pathologists began writing macroscopic (visible to the naked eye) descriptions of endometriosis around this time – referring to menstrual blood in the pelvis and blood-filled growths that may have been endometriomas (endometriosis-filled ovarian cysts).

For the first part of the 19th century, before surgery was commonplace, therapies such as hot douches and morphine were accompanied by more invasive procedures like blood-letting, or the panacea of the 19th century – leeches – applied to the cervix or in the vagina. Caustic substances were also often applied to the cervix, as well as opening the cervix with a dilator, which often led to infection. Even at this stage, when the theory of blood in the pelvis from the period was widely accepted, the idea of a displaced or wandering uterus was still part of the prevailing wisdom.

With the introduction of anaesthetics, surgery became a more feasible option for the treatment for pelvic collections of blood or what were probably endometriomas, but death rates due to sepsis and bleeding were upwards of 70 per cent. The surgical methods involved puncturing cysts, clawing out the lesions by hand and removing them with scissors or blunt instruments. Taking out ovaries and endometriosis-filled ovarian cysts also began to gain traction in the 1900s – but again, the death rates were exceedingly high.

By the end of the 19th century, when both aseptic techniques and anaesthesia had improved, hysterectomies – removing the uterus – began to be thought of as a cure for endometriosis. This was done not only to stop lesions or disease recurring, but also because it was thought that untreated endometriosis might become cancerous.

John Sampson, known as the father of endometriosis, published a landmark paper in 1927 in which he used the word 'endometriosis' for the first time and elegantly described Sampson's theory – that retrograde menstruation leads to endometriosis growths in the pelvis.

The 1960s heralded a huge new step forward in addressing period problems with the advent of the oral contraceptive Pill. The Pill was first introduced for contraception in the face of a growing population problem and also allowed women to control their reproductive lives for the first time. Because contraception was outlawed in many US and Canadian states at the time, the Pill was originally marketed for 'menstrual regulation'. This helped some women with period pain, but the early Pill had significantly more side effects than modern versions. This finally provided an alternative to the surgical approach.

Open surgery to remove lesions and cysts was still the mainstay of treatment until video-assisted keyhole surgery (laparoscopy) was introduced in the late 1970s. This revolutionised endometriosis surgery, as it was less invasive and led to fewer complications. Video also enabled surgeons to identify and excise smaller and smaller lesions, as surgical views could be magnified on a screen.

If lesions were not found, however, the pain was often said to be 'all in the woman's head' or 'perhaps gastrointestinal'. This would either lead to a whole new series of medical investigations, or the woman would be labelled crazy or a 'difficult patient'.

Female healers

Despite the official histories of medicine, women have always been healers. Long before Hippocrates, Ancient Egyptian female physicians and priestesses viewed health and healing as a spiritual–physical continuum and had a tradition of treating people at temples. In pre-modern times, worship of Mother Earth in all her forms as the ultimate creator and giver of life was commonplace. This gave women a power that was revered in early pre-Christian history.

In Greece around the same period, statues of the goddesses Hygieia and Panacea decorated more than 300 healing temples. Female Greek physicians were highly sought after, and in Ancient Rome many female physicians ran busy practices on an equal footing with male doctors.

In the first half of the 12th century, a woman by the name of Trota is thought to have been a physician and chair of the medical school at the University of Salerno in Italy. The *Trotula*, a three-part medical compendium that with much argument is attributed to Trota, included writings on the conditions of and treatments for women. It was used as a reference text for more than 400 years.

While much of the *Trotula* agreed with the idea of the wandering womb – it did not agree that women were simply dysfunctional men. Instead of describing menstrual blood as poisonous or noxious waste, the *Trotula* states: 'First come the flowers, and after, the fruit.' In other words, the menstrual cycle was a continual shedding of flowers each month until such time as a woman bore the fruit of a child.

Around the same time, Hildegard of Bingen, an abbess in a convent – who in modern times is most famous as a composer – wrote about medicine and especially the female body. Her medical texts, although deferential to religion and god, disregarded the idea of women's inferiority to men and instead espoused the view that the natural world and the human body were closely intertwined. Hildegard believed that the earth, the body and the spirit were united aspects of health, and her remedies often included good diet, movement and rest as well as healing herbs. She advocated and encouraged self-healing of patients as a gardener would tend to plants.

Although the earlier account of the history of women and Western medicine is very Anglo/Eurocentric, in many other cultures throughout the world, female healers – including medicine women and shamans – were commonplace.

Wise women were the first healers, herbalists and midwives. They would have worked with nature, encouraging the inner spirit of the patient, rather than attacking disease and hence the body, with powerful and often deadly medicine. From the 10th century onwards, they came into direct opposition with the ever more powerful church and its belief that women's pain and suffering were god's punishment for Eve's original sin – and that such pain and suffering should not be interfered with. The Eve myth is the basis of so-called female inferiority, and its scars still live deep in our bones.

While estimates vary, most historical records indicate that around 50,000 women were killed during the witch hunts in Europe from the 13th to 17th centuries, while a great many others were raped or tortured. Although this sounds like a huge number, it was still only a small part of the population. The efficacy of the strategy was the fear it created. Women did still engage in healing – but in secret. They were pushed outside the mainstream. If women remained submissive, passive and uneducated they were left alone, but if they rebelled they were often destroyed.

The lessons of history
We need to remember this history, because the fear of speaking out, and the hatred and distrust of our own body lives on inside

us. Why is it that a girl hits puberty and begins to feel an inex-plicable shame about her changing body? Why is it that, in the main, we no longer revere and celebrate women's bodies for the wonder that they hold – the power to create and sustain life (as is still done in some traditional cultures around the world)? Why are these very same things that used to imbue us with a mystical power now seen as simply obstacles to success because they make us different from men?

In part it's because of the stories etched into our bones from these times – that women are dysfunctional and shameful, our bodies most of all. We see the messages that reinforce this in our culture all the time. Often even without being aware of the soup we're swimming in, we grow up knowing these things instinctively. Not only do we carry this feeling of not-good-enough and dysfunctionality compared to our brothers, but we also carry the collective trauma of what happened to women all those hundreds of years ago. This sense of collective trauma stays with us even if we can't remember it. It's there when we feel afraid to speak our truth but don't know why. It's there in all the ways we still bow to the patriarchy to keep us safe. It has kept us submissive to a culture in the cleverest and trickiest of ways. It has taught us that we can do anything we want, achieve success in the linear way the patriarchy has defined – if we can only deny our womanhood and female biology. Western medicine can help us with that, of course – it can shut down our cycles, turn off our hormones and prevent the growth, death and rebirth process that occurs within us each month – but at what cost?

Women and modern medicine

The mostly male medical establishment, alongside the church, took over control of the female body. The understanding of the superiority of men as healers, even among women, meant that we stopped handing down knowledge of the body from mother to daughter and instead outsourced that knowledge to authorities outside ourselves. The female body ceased being a wondrous part of nature and become categorised, medicalised and pathologised by a medical system that separated its parts from their function as part of the whole.

It's no accident that many of us feel broken and other, or that we come to anticipate and expect the pain and shame of our monthly periods. It's also no accident that we came to see our saviour in the surgery and drugs of modern medicine. When the Pill came along we became untethered from our natural cycle and our pain was reduced to tiny lesions on a video screen. But if this approach works for you, you become reliant on someone in a position of authority doing something to you again and again. Your power is lost. If it doesn't work – as is often the case – you are left feeling more broken than ever.

We like to think we've come a long way from labelling women hysterical and locking them up in asylums, calling them crazy, telling them their pain is normal and that to be a woman is to suffer. We like to think that modern medicine no longer ignores, dismisses and sometimes actively harms women. After years of working within this paradigm, I have come to believe that our focus on endometriosis lesions as the sole cause of something as complex as pelvic pain is wrong. Pursuing the destruction of a lesion at all costs may be actively harming many women. It creates a culture of fear, disconnection and mistrust of self, and perpetuates the belief that as women we are inherently broken.

The idea that pain is a purely surgical issue is far too simplistic for such a complex concept as pain. It discounts innumerable significant factors that can't be photographed or surgically excised but are as real as, and possibly more important than, an endometriosis lesion.

This book will explain the problem with endometriosis being considered the sole cause of period and pelvic pain and outline all the factors that contribute to the development of pain, particularly the effects of trauma, stress and culture. We will see that the very strategies that have been offered as the solution may well be making the whole problem worse. And I will show you an alternative view that aims to address the whole picture and not just an endometriosis lesion. This book will give you the power to know your own body and give you the tools you need to troubleshoot any problems. We will use what we've learnt from science and the medical model, but in combination with the traditional ways of knowing, of understanding that we are nature and we are not broken – we are whole and perfect.

Chapter summary

- The history of modern medicine and women's pain is one of power and control over, and destruction of, natural processes, as well as the reduction of pain to a physical lesion.
- Women have always had a deep wisdom and reverence of their bodies and cycles as they have in the past for nature.
- There was a time that women were revered for the power to create life and the magical nature of their bodies.
- Women were disconnected from this power by the rise of organised religion and patriarchy and we still hold echoes of this fear and shame in our bodies today, affecting our nervous system and affecting the relationship we have with our bodies.

3

What is endometriosis?

Imagine you've been to the doctor and tried the hormonal drugs with little improvement. The next thing on the doctor's mind – and probably yours, given its increasing profile as the main culprit for pelvic pain – is endometriosis. Your doctor will likely recommend a visit to a gynaecologist, and a laparoscopy to diagnose and treat or exclude endometriosis.

Let's begin by focusing right in on that endometriosis lesion – just as the current medical model does. The standard view is that endometriosis is the main cause of severe period and pelvic pain in women. But what do we really know about endometriosis and its link to pelvic pain, and is the diagnosis and treatment of endometriosis alone effective in treating pelvic pain?

You may be among the one in nine women who have been diagnosed with endometriosis (this figure is based on population data and so the true incidence of endometriosis, given it requires an operation to diagnose, is unknown). Or you could have pelvic pain that's interfering with your life. Or you could simply have a growing awareness of endometriosis as a condition that seems increasingly common, particularly among young women. Most women who come into my office are not exactly sure what endometriosis is. What almost all of them believe, however, is that it causes pain and infertility and requires an operation to diagnose. More often than not, it's associated with a high level of fear – which extends to health practitioners who are unaware of all the factors in the development of chronic pain, only amplifying fear.

In an attempt to not discount women, the current medical paradigm rightly recommends early recognition of severe period pain in women and girls, and in doing so teaches women that the thing to be afraid of and not to miss, is endometriosis. But if, here in Australia at least, there is a push for more and more women to undergo laparoscopic (keyhole) surgeries to diagnose and treat endometriosis, more young women are being commenced on hormonal drugs to switch off the menstrual cycle or reduce bleeding (over a third of young women) and awareness of endometriosis as a dangerous disease in women is at an all-time high, why am I seeing growing numbers of women with severe period pain and progression to persistent pelvic pain despite the recommended treatments?

In the growing consciousness of young women, endometriosis is a dark, nefarious, almost cancer-like condition that always leads to debilitating pain, infertility and chronic disease. The fear of it has seeped into our psyche. Like many things we can't readily see, endometriosis becomes larger and scarier in our mind's eye. So let's start by shedding some light into those dark and scary-seeming corners of our pelvis and look at some facts about endometriosis.

The characteristics of endometriosis

Endometriosis is a term to describe cells found growing outside the uterus that resemble the endometrial cells of the uterine lining. These endometriosis cells occur mostly in the pelvis – often on or around the ovaries, on the surface of the pelvis lining (peritoneum), on the underside of the uterus, and sometimes on the bladder or bowel. The symptoms that lead to an endometriosis diagnosis include period and pelvic pain (which can be chronic or just with periods), bladder or bowel pain, bloating, fatigue, pain with sex and infertility. But some women who have been diagnosed with endometriosis experience no pain or other symptoms. And around half of women who have a laparoscopy to look for endometriosis because of their pelvic pain have no evidence of lesions.

Rarely, endometriosis can be found in other areas of the body such as on the diaphragm and, incredibly rarely, the lungs. Sometimes it can be seen within an abdominal scar, such as a caesarean section scar – in which case it is usually thought to have occurred by contamination with endometrial cells during surgery.

For the purposes of this book, because it is by far and away the most common, we will focus on pelvic endometriosis.

Pelvic endometriosis occurs with varying degrees of severity. In superficial endometriosis, the most common type by far (80 per cent of women with endometriosis) the lesions are clear, red, brown or black deposits that look like tiny freckles on the surface of the peritoneum (the lining of the inside of the pelvis). Think of these as analogous to algae growing on the surface of a pond – they don't send roots down into the surrounding area.

In severe endometriosis, the endometrial cells occur either in the ovaries or can be deep-infiltrating, penetrating deep into surrounding tissues elsewhere in the pelvis – or both. When endometriosis grows within the ovary, it can form endometriomas – ovarian cysts filled with blood, endometrial tissue or old menstrual blood that can look like melted chocolate, giving them their other name, chocolate cysts. Of women diagnosed with endometriosis, 15 per cent have endometriomas and 5 per cent have deep-infiltrating lesions.

In adenomyosis, the endometrial-like cells grow in the muscle layer of the uterus. This is usually diagnosed using an ultrasound or MRI, and is becoming increasingly common due to the increasing sensitivity of scans. Women who have adenomyosis may have heavy or painful periods and may have issues conceiving.

As for endometriosis, though, many women whose scan shows they have adenomyosis don't have any symptoms. This is the paradox of endometriosis and adenomyosis when it comes to pelvic pain.

What causes endometriosis?

The most widely accepted theory as to how most endometriosis cells get into the pelvis is through retrograde menstruation. This occurs when, during a period, some of the blood and endometrial cells pass backwards from the uterus, through the fallopian tubes and into the pelvis. We know that this happens in almost 90 per cent of menstruating women, so the mere presence of those cells in the pelvis cannot be a disease.

Endometriosis lesions occur when those cells start to stick to structures in the pelvis and start to grow where they have landed. We think this is when they may become more of a problem. The most common view is that problems with immune system function contribute to the development of endometriosis, and that at its heart it's a condition of immune system dysregulation. Because endometriosis has rarely been reported in men, in pre-pubertal girls and at distant sites, other theories have also been proposed that may play a part in the development of these rare cases. The other two theories are that extrauterine cells may change into endometrial-like cells (metaplasia) or that endometrial cells are spread via blood or the lymphatic system. While the retrograde menstruation theory is most widely accepted as the most common cause of endometriosis, in some rare cases the development of endometriosis may be multifactorial.

The role of the immune system in endometriosis

It's the immune system's job to recognise the endometrial cells in the pelvis and sweep them up so they don't start to embed. When the immune system becomes dysfunctional, the usual healthy clean-up doesn't occur and instead altered immune cells begin to promote inflammation.

Healthy immune system function is crucial to the way the endometrium sheds and regrows in the uterus each month. One of the key players in the endometriosis immune response is one of our most common immune cells – the macrophage. When functioning correctly, macrophages in our tissues, organs and blood recognise and sweep away pathogens such as viruses and bacteria, and dying and abnormal cells. They also recruit other immune cells and release inflammatory chemicals. During menstruation, macrophages in the uterus help with the breakdown and shedding of the old endometrial lining and in the growth of its replacement. They have oestrogen receptors on their surface, and their number and functions are altered by changing oestrogen levels throughout the cycle.

Within endometriosis lesions, the macrophages appear to have reduced cleaning-up capability but increased inflammatory capability. Instead of removing the endometrial-like tissue in the pelvis, these cells are more likely to make inflammatory chemicals and promote new blood vessel and nerve formation – all of which contribute to the growth and maintenance of endometriosis lesions. Inflammatory responses from mast cells help drive the chronic inflammatory state of endometriosis and the immune cells within an endometriosis lesion become abnormal.

When oestrogen is peaking during the cycle, the endometriosis cells grow, while as oestrogen and progesterone fall before a period, inflammation increases. This process continues and perpetuates the process of inflammation within the endometrial lesion. Endometriosis lesions tend to respond strongly to oestrogen but are more resistant to the inhibitory effects of progesterone.

What triggers endometriosis?

If retrograde menstruation is basically universal, why do some women have a beautiful neat and tidy pelvis, while in others the chaotic and crazy immune system leaves more of a mess? Some women with endometriosis were born with an obstruction in the uterus, cervix or vagina that prevents menstrual flow from the vagina, and so blood and endometrial tissue build up in the pelvis because that's the only direction they can flow. For most of these women, however, removing the obstruction resolves their endometriosis.

The only positive predictive risk factor for endometriosis found at laparoscopy is increasing age, which makes sense as the more periods a woman has the greater the 'wear and tear' from retrograde menstruation.

However, endometriosis does occur in young women and a dysfunctional immune system which impairs the body's ability to clear up these cells is probably the most important factor in the development of severe endometriosis. The most up-to-date theory on what may cause the immune system to become dysregulated, making it ineffective at removing endometriosis cells and instead creating a chronic inflammatory response, is the effect of a bacterial chemical called lipopolysaccharide (LPS). LPS, which is a major component of the outer wall of bacteria such as *E. coli*, can act as a toxin in humans and is a particularly potent activator of the immune system. At this point, let me introduce you to another key player in the endometriosis and pain story: the toll-like receptor (TLR4). LPS binds to TLR4 receptors which are expressed on macrophages (those common immune cells that become dysfunctional in endometriosis) and other immune cells including B-cells, dendritic cells and monocytes. They activate the cells to produce pro-inflammatory chemicals called cytokines, as well as nitric oxide and also induce oxidative stress which drives inflammation. TLR4 cells are implicated in pain conditions with and without endometriosis and are also activated by stress, which is important to remember and we will go into this in detail in Chapters 9 and 10.

We know that the same molecular and cellular processes occur in women with pelvic pain, regardless of the cause.

Bacteria with LPS in their walls are abundant in the human gut and can also live in the vagina – usually due to contamination from the gut. LPS is not bad in itself, but when it interacts with our immune system, problems can arise.

There are two possible theories as to how LPS interacts with immune cells to cause endometriosis. The first is through bacteria in the vagina being taken into the pelvis via retrograde menstruation, activating pelvic and endometrial macrophages along the way.

The second and most likely theory is they come through the gut wall. The wall of the gut is made up of only a single layer of cells, called enterocytes, which are held together like glue by what we call tight junctions. Above this layer of cells is a thick mucous layer, which separates the inside of the intestine – containing the food we eat, chemicals on that food and of course the 9 trillion microbes of our microbiome – from our immune system.

About 70 per cent of our body's immune cells reside just on the other side of that single layer of enterocytes and their protective mucous covering, so the integrity of the mucous and the tight junctions between the enterocytes is crucial. A healthy and diverse gut microbiome helps the cells maintain a healthy mucous layer and protect the enterocytes and the tight junctions, and also contributes to gut wall integrity. The gut microbiome is made up of a balance of beneficial (good guys) and some pathogenic (bad guys) bacteria, and their health and harmony is vital to our human health. Not only can an imbalance of bad and good bacteria make infection more likely, but low microbial diversity – called dysbiosis – can lead to increased inflammation, autoimmune disease, hormonal issues, gastrointestinal symptoms, metabolic problems or weight gain, and even depression.

Research into the gut microbiome has exploded in recent years, and although in many ways we are still at the beginning of learning what's normal and just how integral our gut bacteria are to our overall health, what we do know can help explain the immune system dysfunction of endometriosis.

Research has shown that women with endometriosis often have lower levels of beneficial bacteria called lactobacilli and higher levels of pathogenic or not-so-beneficial bacteria which may lead to higher levels of LPS. This dysbiosis or imbalance can lead to a thinner protective mucous layer and damage to the tight junctions or 'glue' that holds the enterocytes together. If the integrity of the intestinal wall is disturbed, it can lead to increased intestinal permeability or 'leaky gut'. This allows the immune cells to come into contact with pathogens and toxins from the gut, including LPS. These immune cells, such as TLR4, can then migrate to other areas of the body where they are needed – such as the pelvis where they can cause too much inflammation instead of just cleaning up endometriosis cells. TLR4 cells also increase inflammation in the brain which leads to chronic pain. The issue is the studies on microbiome and endometriosis probably don't take into account many women who have endometriosis with no pain – so it may be that women with chronic pain itself have more dysbiosis and thereby more immune dysfunction.

ORIGINS OF PERSISTENT PAIN

There is also recent evidence (albeit in mice), suggesting that endometriosis is more prevalent in mice who were colonised with a particular kind of bacteria (fusobacterium). This study also showed that antibiotic treatment may be effective in reducing lesion size. These findings are yet to be replicated in humans and as we will discover – pain in women is hardly ever just about the presence or absence of an endometriosis lesion. However, it does highlight the importance of the gut microbiome when it comes to immune dysfunction and increased inflammation.

While endometriosis is not classified as an autoimmune disease, in many ways it acts like one, given the inflammatory overreaction to the body's 'own' cells. This gut–immune system connection may also be implicated in several autoimmune diseases, and it is interesting to note that rates of autoimmune disease including lupus, coeliac disease, autoimmune thyroid disease, inflammatory bowel disease and rheumatoid arthritis are higher in women with endometriosis. This may indicate that they occur via a similar pathway.

Are endometriosis lesions always a problem?

Let's zoom out again for a moment and look at the concept of these lesions as always representing disease. Women who have severe disease, with large endometriomas or deep-infiltrating endometriosis, probably represent a subtype of endometriosis which is more likely to be associated with an impaired immune system rather than just the simple wear and tear of periods which is the likely cause in the 80 per cent of women with superficial lesions. Severe and deep endometriosis probably represents those cases described in the history books and are more likely to reflect a true disease state. Even so, there is little correlation between severity of disease and pain or symptoms which again highlights the fact that endometriosis doesn't always equal pain and vice versa.

I would even argue that this superficial endometriosis may not be a disease at all.

Many people think that the presence of an endometriosis lesion is always pathological – meaning indicative of disease – but there's a great deal of evidence that most endometriosis may be physiological – meaning simply part of how our bodies actually work. It may just be a part of a normal menstruating body to have some of these cells in our pelvis at any given time. If bleeding is not too heavy, so that the immune system is not overwhelmed by clean-up work or there is no excessive inflammatory response, these cells can be dealt with efficiently. The mere presence of a lesion at the time of a laparoscopy does not always imply underlying immune system dysregulation. In fact, a study following up women who had no symptoms but were found to have endometriosis at laparoscopy were less likely to report pain than women in the control group who had no endometriosis.

The problem is, if a woman has a laparoscopy for pain and it reveals only mild lesions, she will still be diagnosed with endometriosis – even if her body had it under control and the cells would have been cleaned up by a healthy functioning immune system given half a chance. It's like doing a spot inspection in a rental property to find a mess after a party before the scheduled cleaning day. It's possible that two weeks later the lesions would have been cleaned away.

Does endometriosis always cause pain?

Some studies have reported the presence of endometriosis lesions during routine laparoscopies to tie the fallopian tubes – but these women had no pain. In one of these studies – conducted in the 90s – up to 44 per cent of women with no reported symptoms displayed some endometriosis at laparoscopy. Given the improved sensitivity of laparoscopy equipment, I would guess that this figure would be much higher today. It seems increasingly likely that superficial endometriosis is just part of being a menstruating woman and not a disease process.

It seems logical that if a woman has pelvic pain and when we look inside her pelvis and find lesions with varying degrees of severity, then those lesions must be the cause of the pain – but there is a major flaw in this logic. Until very recently, clinical trials on women have been very rare. The very thing that we need to understand more – our menstrual cycle – is the same thing that historically has precluded women from trials and medical research.

I believe that this means – especially in gynaecology – that we haven't properly established what is actually normal. While a diagnostic laparoscopy is relatively simple in terms of surgery, it's still invasive and comes with risks. This means that apart from the studies on women having their tubes tied, there will never be a randomly selected group of women without pain who will undergo laparoscopy so that we can determine whether it's normal to have endometrial lesions. However, these studies tell us that superficial endometriosis is much more common than we think and if up to almost half of women show evidence of lesions with no symptoms it seems crazy to categorise this as a disease process. Likewise, if up to half of women undergoing laparoscopy have pain but no endometriosis it seems like we need to look for another culprit in what is actually causing pelvic pain.

CASE STUDY: SARAH

Sarah was referred to me by her GP. She was 39, single and was thinking of undergoing fertility treatment with donor sperm to have a baby on her own. She had no history of infertility. In the initial process of doing a fertility workup because she had wanted to access donor sperm, Sarah had a pelvic ultrasound that suggested she had a deep endometriosis nodule in her pouch of Douglas – the area between the bowel and the uterus. It also found a small endometrioma in one of her ovaries. Her GP had diagnosed endometriosis and advised her to see a specialist to discuss treatment – even though at this point she had decided not to pursue a baby for her own reasons so was no longer needing any help with fertility.

Sarah arrived in my office terrified of having surgery. She had read all about endometriosis online and was worried about risks. She was shocked to learn that she had a disease she thought she needed surgery for, especially as she had no symptoms. Sarah had no history of painful periods, painful sex, or painful bowel or bladder.

Sarah is one of many examples of women whose scans shows signs of endometriosis but who've never had any symptoms. She simply didn't need endometriosis surgery or treatment. I've seen women just like Sarah who went down the surgery path and then came to me with chronic pain that they never had before surgery, or with post-operative complications. We need to stop treating the 'lesion' rather than the woman.

CASE STUDY: LELA

Lela was 31 and had recently had her tubes tied as permanent contraception. She was concerned because her surgeon had reported finding superficial endometriosis during her operation. Lela had no concerns about period pain or any other symptoms, but wanted reassurance that she didn't need any other treatment for the endometriosis. In Lela's case, the surgeon had probably found mild 'physiological' endometriosis that her immune system would likely clear up in due course. She did not need surgery or any other treatment, given it was not causing her any problems.

Even with more severe cases of endometriosis, many women experience no pain. While endometriomas, especially if they are large, can be associated with pain or fertility issues, this is not always the case. A retrospective clinical study showed that in women with endometriomas alone with no other peritoneal disease, only 38 per cent had pelvic pain, while more than 61 per cent reported no pain at all. When women with an endometrioma also have deep-infiltrating peritoneal disease, pain is more likely – in one study, up to 85 per cent of women reported pain.

In deep-infiltrating endometriosis the lesions can be found on the peritoneal surfaces, ligaments holding up the uterus, the area under the uterus or ovaries, on the bowel or on the bladder. Because of ongoing inflammation, and scar tissue, blood vessel and nerve tissue formation, these lesions grow roots like a weed – spreading into underlying and surrounding structures and producing sticky inflammatory substances that can cause pelvic structures to adhere together. While women with deep endometriosis often experience more pain than women with superficial lesions, even with deep-infiltrating disease some women may not have any pain symptoms. If they do have pain, though, they are the ones most likely to respond favourably to surgical excision (removal), but remember this is the rarest type of endometriosis representing only about 5 per cent of lesions.

Diagnosis of endometriosis

While the conventional understanding is that laparoscopy is necessary to diagnose endometriosis, both deep endometriosis and ovarian endometriomas – representing around 20 per cent of all women with endometriosis – can be quite reliably diagnosed with specialised transvaginal ultrasound (to an accuracy of up to 93.9 per cent) or MRI (94.8 per cent). If there is any doubt, when used together, accuracy in looking for deep endometriosis can be improved.

Superficial endometriosis cannot easily be diagnosed on an imaging test because it would be like asking an ultrasound or MRI to pick up a freckle or a superficial scratch. In these cases, the current medical paradigm holds that the gold standard of diagnosis is keyhole surgery or laparoscopy. While I agree that women's pain needs to be addressed early to improve quality of life and prevent the development of chronic pain, I don't think that early surgery for women with ongoing pain but no evidence of deep endometriosis or endometrioma is helpful, and I believe the evidence bears this out – especially as we have established that many women have superficial endometriosis with no pain.

A 2020 study looked at laparoscopy findings from 150 women with chronic pelvic pain who had a normal ultrasound and pre-operative examination. Only 20 per cent had evidence of endometriosis, and almost all of it was stage one, the superficial kind least likely to respond to surgical intervention in terms of pain and that may actually be a normal physiological process. The authors concluded that 'women should be informed of the multifactorial nature of chronic pelvic pain and there should be a comprehensive management pathway for these women as proceeding with invasive laparoscopy does not provide additional benefit in the context of risk, cost and long-term wellbeing.' Based on the information we have, I do not think that laparoscopy to diagnose superficial endometriosis in a woman with chronic pain and a normal good-quality scan is necessary or helpful. Treatment of pain is what's important.

Is endometriosis always progressive?

Many gynaecologists will say that surgery is necessary to remove the majority of early or superficial lesions to avoid progression to severe disease. This is a big fear for many women who come to see me. An amalgamation of clinical trials, where laparoscopies were performed six months apart with no surgical removal or other medical intervention, showed that up to 70 per cent of superficial endometriosis either regressed or remained unchanged.

Natural course of endometriosis between first- and second-look laparoscopy in untreated patients.

SOURCE YEAR	Number of patients	Regression	No change	Progression
Thomas And Cooke, 1987	17	9	0	8
Telimaa et al., 1987	12	1	8	3
Mahmood and Templeton, 1990	11	3	1	7
Overton et al., 1994	15	8	3	4
Sutton et al., 1994	24	7	10	7
Harrison And Barry-Kinsella, 2000	43	27	12	4
Abbot et al., 2004	18	4	6	8
Total	140	59 (42%)	40 (29%)	41 (29%)

Adapted from JLH Evers, *Human Reproduction*, 2013:28:2023

Another study did laparoscopies 3 months apart and found that over 42 per cent of women with superficial endometriosis diagnosed at the first laparoscopy had complete resolution by the second when given no treatment. Even deep endometriosis around the rectum and vagina (considered stage four) can be stable, showing no progression when left untreated in up to 90 per cent of cases. So the idea that all endometriosis acts as an aggressive cancer-like growth and if not removed early will always lead to problems is not borne out by the literature.

Endometriosis and fertility

Endometriosis can be associated with difficulty having a baby but MOST women with endometriosis – around 70 per cent, will have no problems with fertility.

There is evidence that removing endometriosis at a laparoscopy in a woman who has trouble getting pregnant can improve natural pregnancy rates and so this is a time when laparoscopy may be appropriate. There is no evidence to support doing laparoscopic surgery prior to IVF for women with superficial, deep or ovarian endometriosis and surgery should be reserved for those with infertility and pain. Current evidence suggests that pregnancy rates with IVF for women with and without endometriosis are similar.

Chapter summary

- Endometriosis is the presence of endometrial-like cells in the pelvis or areas of the body other than the lining of the uterus.
- Most endometriosis is superficial and may represent part of the normal menstruation process of blood going back into the pelvis through the tubes. **For this reason, early diagnosis becomes less relevant than early treatment of pain.**
- When more severe, endometriosis appears to be a disease of immune dysregulation and over-inflammation. Although, chronic pain without endometriosis also has evidence of immune dysregulation.
- Increased inflammation and pain, regardless of endometriosis, is associated with LPS activation of a special immune cell

(TLR4) that lives between the immune and nervous system which amplifies pain and brain inflammation.

- Most endometriosis either stays the same or gets better without treatment.
- Many women have endometriosis with no pain and many women have pain with no endometriosis.
- Most women with endometriosis can achieve pregnancy.
- Surgery can diagnose endometriosis and remove lesions but may not improve pain.
- **Laparoscopy should not be first-line management for chronic pelvic pain in the presence of a normal good-quality ultrasound or MRI.**

4

The pharmaceutical approach to endometriosis

The days of ignoring women's physical pain is thankfully over. Medical practitioners, parents, and women and girls themselves are aware of the need to treat pain promptly in order to avoid the development of long-term pain. Social media is allowing women to tell their stories and raise awareness at a grassroots level. Pelvic pain, but more importantly the idea of endometriosis as the leading cause of pain in women, has gained massive momentum – which, as you can see from the last chapter, is deeply flawed.

The approach that I was taught as a gynaecologist in training many years ago is not all that different from the current approach to managing pelvic pain. Most women are taught that if their pain is severe, lasts throughout the entirety of the period, or interferes with their ability to carry on as usual – missing days of school, work or other activities – then the pain may be due to endometriosis, which may require turning off periods with hormonal medications or an operation.

Most GPs or gynaecologists will initially advise painkillers/anti-inflammatories such as ibuprofen or Ponstan (mefenamic acid). If these aren't effective, they will suggest a hormonal option to reduce bleeding and inflammation associated with a period or simply take periods away all together. These hormonal approaches include the Pill, hormonal IUDs, Depo Provera implants and even turning off the body's reproductive hormones with a drug to make a woman temporarily menopausal. If these treatments aren't effective in three to six months, the next step is often laparoscopic surgery to look for and remove endometriosis. Although this is not how I practise any more, this is still very much the status quo when it comes to primary care of pelvic pain – especially as the call for early diagnosis of endometriosis becomes louder.

The Pill is far and away the most common starting point for women who visit their GP with pelvic pain. The aim is to reduce bleeding in order to reduce inflammation, and this does reduce pain for many women. It's important, however, to look at just how the Pill and other hormonal approaches work, how they affect endometriosis and how they affect the rest of the woman.

The Pill

The Pill or combined oral contraceptive Pill, works by basically turning the reproductive system off at the level of the brain, switching off our own production of oestrogen, progesterone and testosterone, and replacing our natural ovarian hormones with a blend of synthetic oestrogen and progestin. It also stops ovulation, which is why it's used as a contraceptive drug. This changes the ebbs and flows of a natural cycle to a flat line of oestrogen and progestin with no testosterone. A period, by definition, occurs around two weeks after ovulation and is the release of an unfertilised egg and the subsequent shedding and rebuilding of the endometrium (the lining of the uterus) to start again the following month. Most types of Pill have 21–24 days of active or hormone tablets followed by 4–7 days of sugar pills. Taking the sugar pills mimics our natural fall in hormones at the end of a cycle and brings on a withdrawal bleed – the uterine lining needs constant hormone levels to remain stable, and if they fall it stimulates the shedding response. This is not a period – as ovulation didn't occur – it's just a shedding of the lining in response to an artificial hormone drop.

If this bleed is artificial and we're making it happen by choosing to take the sugar pills, then we can choose not to take the sugar pills and just continue with the active hormonal tablets. In this case a bleed does not occur and women can 'skip' bleeds for several months or choose when it's convenient for them to have a bleed.

An interesting fact is that when the Pill was invented in the 1960s, the decision was made to put sugar pills in so that the women taking it would still feel like they had a period. It was an effort to make the Pill feel more 'natural' to women, to assure them they weren't pregnant and to appease the Catholic Church. To this day, many women still think that the bleed that comes with sugar pills is a real period or that the Pill 'regulates' their cycle. But the Pill turns the cycle off, whether or not you bleed. For this reason, 'skipping' a bleed on the Pill is not harmful and can help many women with painful periods.

The Pill can definitely improve pain symptoms, usually by making the uterine lining thinner and therefore resulting in reduced bleeding, or by allowing women to skip their bleeds altogether. This reduces the amount of normal inflammatory chemicals called prostaglandins that are released as the endometrium sheds and also at ovulation.

The Pill can have several side effects and risks. It's important for your doctor to discuss these with you so that you can make an informed decision.

The risks of the Pill

Most doctors will tell you that when you take the Pill there's a slightly higher risk of venous thromboembolism (blood clots in a leg vein that can also move to the lungs). The risk is small: 7–10 per 10,000 women studied over one year compared to 2 per 10,000 in women not taking the Pill. To put it in perspective, women have an almost 30 in 10,000 risk of blood clots during pregnancy. The rate of arterial thrombosis (a blood clot in an artery) is about 1.6 times higher in women taking the Pill than those who aren't.

Breast cancer risks are only slightly increased on the Pill. For every 100,000 women not taking the Pill, 55 will get breast cancer each year compared to 65 women taking the Pill. Cervical cancer rates in women taking the Pill are very slightly increased. On the other hand, rates of endometrial and ovarian cancer are decreased in women taking the Pill for a long time – the benefit is greatest over 10 years. This still only means, however, that roughly 185 women would need to take the Pill for more than five years in order to prevent one case of ovarian or endometrial cancer.

Possible side effects of the Pill

It's important to point out that not all women who take the Pill will suffer side effects, and if they do, they generally won't experience all of them. Most women are never told about the possibility of these side effects, and even though many will be fine, they should still be properly informed.

The reality is, many women who end up suffering some of these side effects are dismissed and told that it's not the Pill and must be something else. You should always have your symptoms taken seriously so you can experiment and work out what feels right for you – especially when there are many more options for painful periods than just the Pill.

While for some women the Pill can be life-changing for managing painful periods, it shouldn't be the default. It should definitely come with an exploration of the root cause of the pain, and a proper discussion about how the Pill works, its potential side effects and other options.

Common side effects that we often hear about are weight gain, bloating, headaches, breast tenderness and irregular bleeding. Other side effects can include mood changes – depression, anxiety or just not feeling like yourself.

Mood changes

Studies on the effect of the Pill on mood are mixed, but a recent large Danish study involving more than 1 million women reported that Pill users were 1.2 times more likely to be prescribed an antidepressant than non-users and in younger women this increased to 1.8 times. Research has also shown that starting the Pill in adolescence, at a time where the brain is organising itself and particularly vulnerable to the influences of hormones such as oestrogen, progesterone and testosterone, could cause possibly irrevocable developmental changes in the way the brain is unorganised.

I often see women who were commenced on the Pill quite soon after their first period and have remained on it for many years. When they do come off the Pill, these women often struggle from a mood point of view, as their brains have to get used to the natural ups and downs of hormones in a natural cycle. Getting used to hormones is one of the reasons why the teenage years are often thought of as a dramatic, crazy rollercoaster. It can be hard for young women to adjust to the cyclical nature of their body and their hormones, as many parents can attest. If we rob women of that initiation, we essentially create an artificial environment with no cyclical ebbs and flows and give them no opportunity to learn the language of their body. This can result in women who are unable to function off the Pill in later life, or to cope with the hormonal changes at menopause, because their brains have not become resilient to hormone fluctuations and can only tolerate a constant hormone level.

The Pill's effects on mood are thought to be mostly due to it preventing our ovaries from making their own progesterone and replacing it with synthetic progestins. Unlike synthetic progestins, natural progesterone converts into a hormone called allopregnanolone that activates receptors in the brain to have a calming, soothing effect. When you take the Pill, which stops you from ovulating, you miss out on your monthly dose of calming allopregnanolone.

Loss of testosterone

The Pill stops the ovaries from making testosterone, which is the hormone of confidence and agency as well as (alongside oestradiol) a driver of sexual desire. In addition, pills containing oestrogen switch on the production in the liver of a protein called sex hormone binding globulin (SHBG), which further reduces the circulating testosterone by mopping up the testosterone produced by the adrenal glands. Reduced circulating testosterone may be why the Pill often causes women to experience a decrease in libido. A recent Australian study also reported that women on the Pill have lower motivation – particularly that they lose the mid-cycle drive that comes with the elevation of testosterone and oestrogen. Many women report feeling 'numb' or 'more level' – which can be welcome for some, but takes the colour out of life for others.

The lack of testosterone, while effective for treating acne, can also have an effect on the vaginal and vulval skin in some women. The vulva has testosterone receptors and needs testosterone and oestradiol to be healthy. Without this some women can develop thin, sensitive vulval skin, which can lead to pain during sex. Some new research also suggests that women with low testosterone levels may experience higher pain perception than those with higher levels. Ironically, while many women are put on medications for painful periods, their effect on hormone levels may contribute to increased persistent pain.

Bone density

While a 2014 Cochrane review (i.e. one that aggregates the best-quality medical studies) found that the Pill had no significant effect on bone density, a recent 2018 meta-analysis (i.e. one that merges several smaller studies to look for overall effects) showed that young women who take the Pill may have lower bone density. This may be important given that many women start the Pill as teenagers and are on it for many years.

Metabolism

The Pill has also been associated with nutritional and other metabolic changes. It can cause elevation of triglycerides (blood fats) and a decline in glucose tolerance (a step towards type 2 diabetes). This is important because many women with polycystic ovarian syndrome (PCOS) and impaired glucose tolerance are put on the Pill to regulate their cycle and drive down testosterone. Unless they also make changes to their diet and lifestyle, the Pill could potentially worsen their insulin resistance.

Fertility

Most women's fertility returns to normal when they go off the Pill, but sometimes it can take months for periods to return if the hypothalamus (the master controller of all the hormones in the body) is particularly sensitive and the brain and ovaries take a longer time to restart the conversation they were having before the Pill. This is particularly true if girls are started on the Pill very early after their first period. It takes around eight years for the reproductive system to reach full maturity, and for many women up to two years for their natural cycle to become regular – which means regular ovulation.

I often explain the brain and ovary connection as like your body learning an amazing new skill. If we were to pick up the violin one day and start to play, most of us would be terrible at it. The same is true for our reproductive system. If we start the Pill while our periods are still irregular, it's akin to taking the violin out of our hands because we're not very good yet and putting a Spotify mix of a master violinist on. Suddenly it's perfect. Pill bleeds are regular – and give the illusion of a perfect cycle – but in reality there is no cycle and no ovulation. The Pill essentially prevents the reproductive system from practising at ovulation, and so it's stuck in the same state it was when the Pill was started. If your periods aren't regular when you start the Pill, it's not uncommon for them to be irregular when you come off it later in life. It's like stopping the Spotify mix 10 years later and asking you to start playing the violin again. You still won't be very good because you haven't practised.

This can be a problem for many women – particularly if they come off the Pill in order to fall pregnant. While the Pill can be a big help for young women with heavy or painful periods, they need to know that if the root cause is never addressed, they might simply be kicking the can down the road – only to deal with the same issue years later or be pushed into the pipeline of fertility treatments.

Progestin-only pills: Slinda, Visanne and Provera

While the combined oral contraceptive Pill contains both oestrogen and progestin, some other pills containing only progestin are often used for pain and endometriosis. Because endometriosis, like the endometrium (uterine lining), is stimulated to grow by oestrogen – like fertiliser for a lawn – and that growth is inhibited by progesterone or progestin, these progestin-only pills may help with endometriosis and/or pain by reducing bleeding and by reducing growth of the lesions themselves.

Drospirenone (sold as Slinda) is a synthetic progestin that works by turning off ovulation and stopping the ovaries from producing oestrogen and progesterone. It also works directly on the lining of the uterus to thin it, which reduces uterine shedding and bleeding considerably. As it stops ovulation, most women will not have a proper period and thus, as with the combined Pill, it reduces inflammation related to bleeding.

Dienogest (sold as Visanne) is another progestin-only drug marketed for pelvic pain and endometriosis. It works to suppress the growth of endometrial and endometriosis cells, but is not licensed for contraception as it may not reliably suppress ovulation.

Medroxyprogesterone acetate (sold as Provera) is a synthetic progestin that suppresses the lining of the uterus and potentially ovulation – depending on the dose. Provera is often suggested long-term to reduce bleeding and decrease the growth of endometriosis.

Depo Provera is an injectable version of Provera that lasts for three months and works by suppressing ovulation and hence hormones. Because it's quite a high dose, side effects such as weight gain and mood changes are more likely.

Implanon is a rod-shaped implant inserted under the skin in the upper arm which contains a synthetic progestin. While it is excellent for contraception, I never use it in clinical practice, especially not for pain or bleeding because there is a 40 per cent risk of ongoing and unpredictable bleeding which doesn't decrease with time.

The risks of progestin-only treatments

Fertility can take up to 18 months to come back on line after ceasing Depo Provera injections. There is also a risk of bone loss or osteoporosis with long-term Depo Provera use. It's a misnomer to only call oestrogen and our other ovarian hormones reproductive or sex hormones, because they have effects on the whole body. Bone health and strength are related to oestrogen and progesterone levels – without sufficient oestrogen there may be an increased risk of bone loss or osteoporosis, but the long-term effects of progesterone-only drugs on bone density have not yet been studied.

Possible side effects of progestin-only treatments

Side effects of progestin-only medications can be similar to those of the combined Pill – mood changes, weight gain, breast tenderness, headaches and irregular bleeding or spotting. Unlike the Pill, however, they don't cause an increase in blood-clot risk because they don't contain oestrogen.

This is a good thing on one hand, particularly for women whose other conditions make the Pill ill advised, but the omission of oestrogen can lead to other problems. When the ovaries aren't making oestrogen because of suppression caused by these drugs and it's not being replaced with a synthetic version – oestrogen levels are low. While this reduces menstrual bleeding and potentially endometriosis growth, oestrogen has important functions outside our pelvis.

When the ovaries aren't making progesterone it can affect mood, as synthetic progestin doesn't have the same calming effect as the natural progesterone we only make after ovulation. Without oestrogen to increase serotonin in the brain, there can be a double-whammy effect on mood. All hormonal drugs have the capacity to have an effect on the brain and some women are more sensitive to the potentially negative effects of progestin than others.

Lack of oestrogen and testosterone can also affect libido and potentially cause the vulval and vaginal thinning that we saw with the combined Pill.

These drugs can be used alone but are also often prescribed on top of other hormonal drugs, such as the hormonal IUD.

It is interesting to note that while many doctors tell women, particularly if they have been diagnosed with endometriosis, that they need to stay on some form of synthetic progestin to 'stop endometriosis growing back', the evidence for this is lacking. A study that carried out a laparoscopy on women with endometriosis and infertility gave half the women Provera and half the women a placebo and did a re-look laparoscopy 3 months later. They found that both the placebo and Provera were as effective as each other at reducing endometriosis lesions with the placebo arm showing a 42 per cent complete resolution of endometriosis at the second laparoscopy! This shows again that endometriosis can ebb and flow and resolve on its own and that synthetic progestin was no better than a placebo at reducing the growth of endometriosis.

The hormonal IUD

The Mirena IUD is a small T-shaped device containing a synthetic progestin called levonorgestrel that thins the lining of the uterus. The hormonal IUD is like having a little lawn mower inside the uterus keeping the grass trimmed extra short like a lawn-tennis court. Because it provides a constant dose of progestin in the uterus with no dips, bleeding is much reduced or stops altogether. It is a contraceptive but is also licensed for use in heavy bleeding and period pain. The Kyleena is the Mirena's little sister – it's slightly smaller, contains a lower dose of the progestin, and is often recommended for younger women who have not had children and thus have a smaller uterus.

These IUDs work like the progestin-containing pills – but this time by directly inhibiting the growth of the uterus lining to make periods very light or non-existent for up to 90 per cent of women. This effect usually lasts for three to five years, although it can be contraceptive for up to eight years.

After three to six months, the Mirena (or Kyleena) does not routinely suppress ovulation because the progestin it contains mainly exerts its effect locally. In this way it's quite different from the Pill which completely switches off the ovaries. The Mirena usually allows the ovaries to continue making oestradiol, progesterone and testosterone, and the brain and ovaries keep talking to each other and making and releasing eggs in the background, even though most women won't get a regular period. For this reason, fertility returns to normal almost as soon as the Mirena is removed, and if a Kyleena or Mirena is inserted when a young girl's reproductive system is still maturing, it does not stop her brain and ovaries communicating or practising ovulation. Although the Mirena lasts for 5 to 7 years for contraception, many women with pain may require replacement between 2 and 4 years because of falling hormone levels, to maintain a thin endometrial lining. You will know it may need replacing earlier if you start to have more problematic bleeding.

The risks of hormonal IUDs

The risk of infection from IUDs is very low, less than one in 1000. Your doctor will usually test for any STIs before insertion, to ensure the risk remains low. Perforating the uterus or migration of the Mirena into the pelvis is also very rare, occurring in less than one in 1000 insertions. Occasionally the Mirena may fall out or become mispositioned, which often results in pain or abnormal bleeding. It's easily remedied by removing it and inserting a new Mirena.

Possible side effects of hormonal IUDs

The Mirena can cause some cramping, but this usually dissipates within the first few days. The other most common side effect of the Mirena is that it usually causes some light unpredictable bleeding for the first few months after insertion.

As with any hormonal contraceptive, some women can experience significant hormonal side effects. Only one-tenth of the progestin dose can be measured in the blood, so blood hormone levels are very low, but some women who are sensitive to the hormone may experience side effects such as acne, hair loss, breast tenderness, bloating or mood changes, and weight gain is uncommon.

Studies on the impact of Mirena on mood and rates of depression and anxiety are mixed. One large 2016 Finnish study of young women using the Mirena showed a higher association (not causation) with depression than in those on the Pill, along with a slightly increased use of antidepressants. A recent meta-analysis showed variable results but confirmed that just like other hormonal drugs, women do report mood changes on the Mirena. These studies have many limitations, of course, and my number one guide is to listen to each woman sitting in front of me and believe what she's feeling in her body.

While some women may be supersensitive to even tiny levels of circulating progestin, I think the most likely reason for mood changes with a Mirena or Kyleena is that the level of hormone is highest just after insertion. This means it's most likely to suppress ovulation for the first few months, and without ovulation we get no mood-boosting effects of oestrogen and testosterone, and no calming effects of natural progesterone. If this is you and the IUD is helping with pain, before giving up on it I suggest asking your doctor to check your hormone levels. If your oestrogen is low, they could prescribe some natural oestrogen for a few months while the concentration of hormone in the Mirena dissipates and ovulation returns.

The strings from the Mirena sit just below the cervix and you can usually only feel them if you felt for them, like removing a tampon. Most partners are unable to feel the strings during sex, but if they do, your doctor may just need to trim the strings a little.

Insertion of IUDs

If you're sexually active, insertion can take place in the doctor's office, but if you're not sexually active, have experienced trauma or simply feel too worried about how you will cope, it can be done under general anaesthesia. The insertion itself takes around five minutes and can range from a little uncomfortable to painful depending on the woman and the insertion. Make sure you feel comfortable with your doctor and take a support person.

In my practice, I find that relaxing music, some breath work before and essential oils to ground you in your body all help, but it's important to talk with your care provider about the things that most help you to feel at ease and safe. Many women find Mirena insertion a traumatic event – on top of other traumas where they found themselves with no control or no voice. It doesn't have to be this way. It can be empowering and you can feel in control if you work with a gentle practitioner who knows your past and is trauma-informed (i.e. understands how trauma affects the body and behaviour, and works hard not to retraumatise through treatment).

GnRH agonists: Zoladex

This drug is usually used as a last resort for severe cases of endometriosis and chronic pain. In my practice I hardly ever use it for the pain of endometriosis because chronic pain is seldom only about endometriosis. GnRH agonists are given once a month as injections just under the skin of the abdomen. They act on the brain at the level of the hypothalamus (your hormone CEO) and work by stopping the brain communicating with the ovaries and thus turning off the reproductive system. It's a little like the Pill but without adding back extra hormones. It can make women feel temporarily menopausal, with side effects such as hot flushes, depression and other mood issues and lowered libido. Long-term effects on the body include lowered bone density, and detrimental effects on metabolism, the heart and cognition. For this reason, GnRH agonists are usually only recommended for six months. Because they turn off the production of oestrogen and ovulation, they stop periods and starve growth of the uterine lining and endometriosis lesions.

This medication does usually improve symptoms associated with endometriosis and obviously reduces any degree of period pain because it turns off periods – but its significant side effects can have a huge influence on quality of life, making it unsustainable in the long term without adding back hormones. A novel drug called Ryeqo, containing an oral form of a GNrH antagonist plus oestrogen and progestin, is just being introduced into the market. While not yet licensed for endometriosis and pain, it works similarly to Zoladex plus hormone add back to turn off the cycle and add-back hormones to reduce side effects. This is also contraceptive after a month and may be another option for women with pelvic pain and/or endometriosis who are wanting to suppress their cycles and reduce the inflammation associated with periods.

It's not uncommon for me to see women who have had two Mirenas inserted (despite the lack of evidence that two are more effective than one), plus the Pill or extra progestin tablets and a course of Zoladex, with several surgeries thrown in for good measure in the relentless pursuit of stopping any bleeding and reducing the growth of endometriosis lesion. While this approach might be helpful for some women, studies on the effect of quality of life and reduction of pain, rather than just the size of endometriosis lesions, are limited.

While I do think it sometimes has a role to play prior to surgery for severe disease, I barely ever use Zoladex for pelvic pain in my practice because other therapies which address the whole woman and not just the hormones and periods are usually far more effective with less side effects.

A meta-analysis on medical treatments and pelvic pain showed that up to 19 per cent of women report no change in symptoms at all and up to 60 per cent still have pain when looking at a mix of all the hormonal treatments. Many women discontinue due to side effects.

CASE STUDY: KATIE

Katie was 31 when she came to me with her husband after undergoing treatment for endometriosis for several years. She felt broken, and while she was hopeful there was another way, she felt sicker than when she had first sought help.

Her sister had recently been diagnosed with endometriosis, but while Katie sometimes had painful periods, they were quite manageable. After her sister's diagnosis, her gynaecologist recommended that Katie also seek a diagnosis, as endo-metriosis often runs in families. Katie went to see her sister's doctor and was promptly booked in for a laparoscopy. Mild endometriosis was diagnosed and two Mirena IUDs were placed. Katie had more pain after the surgery than she had before – her pain was now constant and she had continual bleeding. She was then placed on extra progestin in the form of Provera tablets. This did help to reduce bleeding, but her pain continued.

Katie gained almost 30 kilograms in about six months and became depressed. Her gynaecologist started her on an antidepressant to treat the mood issues caused by all the synthetic progestin. The antidepressant probably contributed to further weight gain. Katie also developed acne that she'd never had before as a side effect of the progestins.

Her pain continued despite these measures, so the Mirenas were eventually removed. When Katie saw me she was not bleeding – and was on the combined Pill plus extra progestin. According to her doctor, her endometriosis was being treated. If she was not bleeding and not ovulating, then the hope was that her endometriosis was being kept at bay. Despite this, her pain continued. She came to me because her doctor's next step was a repeat laparoscopy to look for and remove endometriosis – within two years of her original surgery. Something about this didn't feel right to Katie.

On the one hand she felt like her body had betrayed her – as if she was so dysfunctional and sick that the only way it could be 'managed' was with all these treatments that felt like nuclear bombs to her system. On the other hand, she knew something didn't feel right. The cure should not be worse than the disease. Only she had been told that the disease was dangerous, that it could progress, cause ongoing pain and infertility. But when her pain was worse after the treatment and she had no history of infertility so far, it made her wonder . . . This treatment approach felt wrong. It wasn't improving her pain, it was producing new symptoms and her quality of life had declined.

She was right to doubt.

While hormonal treatments may help many women with symptoms, using them to treat an actual or potential endometriosis lesion can end up burning down the house you're trying to save. Endometriosis is far from the only cause of pelvic pain, and it's caused by more than just hormonal issues. Even if it were true that endometriosis always caused pain, its eradication at the expense of the woman's mental and metabolic health *without actually reducing pain* is not only insane but goes against the doctors' Hippocratic oath: First do no harm. We're supposed to be treating a whole woman and improving her health and quality of life, not merely aiming to treat a lesion by destroying the woman.

Katie came off all her hormone medications and her antidepressant. She felt like a cloud had lifted. We began to deal with all the factors associated with the development of endometriosis, as well as identifying and addressing the other components in her pain picture.

She felt more like herself, started to lose weight, and was able to manage her periods without hormones. She tried to conceive naturally for six months or so, but her ovulation was irregular (not a symptom of endometriosis) – possibly affected by long-term hormonal suppression or by the metabolic effects of all the medications she had been taking. Katie went on to have an IVF cycle and happily conceived after her second embryo transfer.

Seeing Katie learn to love and trust the wisdom of her body and enjoy life again was so rewarding. I see women like Katie every day. Women who feel as if their body has betrayed them, who haven't learnt about the wonders of their body or how to live in harmony with it to increase their chances of good health. They think they need rescuing, but often their rescuer becomes a tormenter and they feel more confused than ever, not knowing who to trust.

Time for a paradigm shift

When we grow up absorbing the idea that female-ness is troublesome, only causing pain, embarrassment, mess and inconvenience, of course we trust someone who tells us that if they turn off our hormones, we'll somehow be saved. Without those pesky hormones, we'll no longer be at the mercy of our wild cyclical nature. The dysfunctionality and unpredictability of our female bodies will be quelled, but often at the expense of our connection to ourselves. When we doctors aren't transparent about the possible side effects of hormonal medications, we are lying to women.

In 1970, in the first decade of the Pill, a US senator, Gaylord Nelson, called for congressional hearings into the potential dangers of the Pill. At the time of the Nelson Pill hearings, the Pill had been approved by the US Food and Drug Administration (FDA) for several years and marketed as a treatment for menstrual disorders – although it was most commonly used for contraception. Many doctors were concerned about the seemingly high number of adverse incidents among women taking the Pill – such as blood clots in the legs or lungs that could be fatal, and severe mood disturbances including an increase in suicide. The fact that the Pill can cause mood disturbances has been debated for years, with some studies concluding it has no such effect – much to the chagrin of women everywhere who have experienced changes in mood.

The hearings concluded – after evidence from doctors, and from scientists in the fields of pharmacology, biology and population control – that the 'potential harm to the individual woman could be outweighed by the benefits to the society and population control as a whole'. Someone even suggested during the hearings that if you counselled women about all the potential risks and side effects of the Pill they would be unlikely to take it.

The result was that the Pill became the first medication to have its potential side effects printed on an insert in the packet. But we know that human nature is such that even if we read these inserts, we tend to trust the prescribing doctor that it will be safe.

Don't get me wrong. The Pill has been an essential part of the feminist movement and the liberation of women, allowing women the reproductive freedom to pursue tertiary education and a career, as well as sexual freedom. It was a game changer. Without it and the positive effects it has had on the women of my generation, as well as my mother's and grandmother's generations, I might not have been able to get a medical degree, open my own practice or feel free in the expression of my views to write this book. While the Pill certainly has its place in modern gynaecology, helping some women with gynaecological symptoms and being a hugely liberating part of women's fight for equality, this story illustrates the lack of informed consent about all the facts for women to make their own minds up. It is a different time now and women deserve the chance to have an informed discussion about the pros and the potential cons of taking the Pill as well as the alternatives. Continuing to use it as a panacea for period problems without looking for the root cause of the issue and without educating women about their bodies is lazy medicine.

As a training gynaecologist I was taught to take a woman's blood pressure before starting her on the Pill, check that she had no personal history or family history of blood clots, and advise her of the tiny increased chance of blood clots, but explain that the risks of a blood clot in pregnancy are much higher than for a woman on the Pill. We weren't taught to discuss a potential change in mood, loss of libido, weight gain or the possibility of painful sex, and we absolutely weren't taught to tell women about the benefits of a natural cycle. But by withholding information from women that would help them make a fully informed decision about what's right for their own body, we're infantilising them.

It may sound like I'm against hormonal drugs. I'm not. However, I do believe that if a woman chooses one of the hormonal drug options she should know the possible side effects. And if it doesn't end up being right for her, that her doctor should support her and discuss alternatives. Many women with endometriosis get told they must be on hormonal drugs to reduce the risk of their endometriosis getting worse or recurring after surgery. But as we will soon see, this is not true for every woman. Many women with endometriosis choose a non-hormonal path and do well. Even a high-quality Cochrane review concluded that there is minimal evidence that the Pill is effective for pain in women with period pain and endometriosis. There is also direct evidence that 3 months of synthetic progestin had the same effect as placebo on endometriosis lesions.

The cure should not be worse than the disease. If you're taking hormonal drugs and your quality of life is improved, that's wonderful. But if it's worse due to side effects, you need to rethink your treatment plan. There's no reason to take hormonal drugs that are making you feel worse simply to treat endometriosis. I've seen women who have been on the Pill for almost the whole of their reproductive lives but still have severe endometriosis. As we are discovering, hormones are not the only driver of endometriosis and pelvic pain and superficial endometriosis may have less to do with pain than we have been led to believe.

Chapter summary

- Hormonal drugs used to suppress periods can help many women with period pain as they reduce the inflammation associated with ovulation and periods.
- It is important to understand how these drugs work as well as all the potential benefits, side effects and risks to help you make an informed decision about the right treatment for you.
- If you have been diagnosed with endometriosis, you don't have to be on hormonal drugs – it is one option for the treatment of pain associated with periods but isn't necessary, especially if you are experiencing more negative side effects than benefits.

5

The surgical approach to endometriosis

As we have seen, the evidence that surgery to remove endometriosis is effective at treating pain is poor at best. Up to half of women who have their lesions excised (removed) surgically, even if their pain initially improves, have a recurrence and resort to further excision removal surgeries. A repeat surgery that finds and removes even one or two more lesions of superficial endometriosis or adhesions is deemed a success, even if the woman will experience very little improvement in pain from this. Surgery is how the healthcare system (hospitals and individual doctors) generate income. For example, Medicare in Australia will rebate a gynaecologist $780 for doing a basic laparoscopy to remove a tiny spot of endometriosis, the anaesthetist around $200 for putting that patient to sleep and the private health fund will pay the hospital around $2000 for the admission. On the other hand, Medicare will rebate a gynaecologist $95.10 for an initial appointment and $46.15 to have a follow-up consultation to discuss and treat the multitude of other factors that contribute to pelvic pain.

I was trained to offer a diagnostic laparoscopy for pain and to claim fees for excision and hormonal therapies as the mainstay of treatment. But I became frustrated at the inadequacy of surgery as a cure for pain. I believe that any surgeon working within this system knows this to be true.

Does surgery improve pelvic pain?

There have only been three randomised controlled trials (RCT) on whether the excision of endometriosis improves pain. RCTs are thought to be the gold standard for evidence-based medicine. This means that participants are randomly assigned to laparoscopy to remove lesions or a diagnostic laparoscopy – no removal of lesions. Only one of these studies was blinded which means that in 2 of 3 studies women knew if they were having lesions removed or not. In one blinded Australian RCT, a small number of women with pain was randomly divided into two groups. All women had a laparoscopy, but the surgeons only excised the endometriosis in one group. They found that pain improved in 80 per cent of women who had endometriosis excised, compared with 32 per cent of those who had the laparoscopic incisions but no endometriosis removed. That's still a placebo effect of over 30 per cent. We know that the placebo effect is amplified the larger the intervention. For example, an injection is likely to create a larger placebo effect than a pill, and a surgery the largest of all. While an 80 per cent improvement in pain is significant, longer term follow-up of this study found that up to 36 per cent of women experienced worsening pain within five years.

After six months, the researchers operated again, this time to excise the endometriosis in the women who'd had the sham surgery the first time. The endometriosis was unchanged or partly or fully resolved in 55 per cent of cases, meaning it had only become worse in about 45 per cent.

A review article looking at the results of all these RCTs, showed the absolute benefit in short-term pain improvement taking into account the large placebo effect for surgery was only 30–40 per cent, with pain recurrence and re-operation rate of up 50 per cent over years. When all these studies were reviewed together it was found that up to 70 per cent of lesions at the 6-month re-operation point were unchanged or improved. This shows again that endometriosis is not always progressive – it's dynamic, and a body in a healthy immunological and hormonal state has the capacity to deal with it.

The Cochrane database collects all the best available evidence to increase the numbers in research and thereby the likelihood of a meaningful answer. A 2020 systematic Cochrane review of laparoscopic surgery for endometriosis concluded that: 'Compared to diagnostic laparoscopy only, it's uncertain whether laparoscopic surgery reduces overall pain associated with minimal to severe endometriosis.' It should also be noted that almost all of the studies comparing diagnostic laparoscopy with excisional surgery have been deemed to be at high risk of bias and classified as low quality and there was no breakdown in these studies as to the effectiveness of surgery on superficial vs deep endometriosis. All endometriosis was lumped together which makes it difficult to determine for whom surgery is most beneficial.

If we are to put all our faith in evidence-based medicine, then this is a blow to the current paradigm that uses surgery to remove endometriosis in order to fix pain. Just as women need to know the score with hormonal treatments for endometriosis and pelvic pain, they need to be counselled with the evidence for surgery so that they have realistic expectations about their chances of pain improvement.

While the effects of surgery on pain and quality of life have likely been overplayed, and while it may not add anything significant to your diagnosis if you've had good-quality scans, when might surgery be appropriate and most likely be beneficial?

Studies tell us that women with cyclical symptoms (pain with their periods, symptoms such as pain with sex *and* who have deep-infiltrating disease are most likely to have positive outcomes with surgery, up to 83 per cent reporting improved or resolved symptoms in the short term. While surgery may be appropriate for this type of endometriosis *if* there are symptoms, there is still a 5–10 per cent risk of bowel, bladder or nerve damage with surgery – depending on the location of the lesion – so the potential improvement to quality of life must always be weighed up against the potential risks of surgery.

On the other hand, women with chronic pelvic pain are only likely to have improved symptoms after surgery 30–40 per cent of the time – and this is without considering long-term recurrence of symptoms, which can be as high as 50 per cent.

Repeat surgery for pain is also likely to be a game of diminishing returns, with most evidence pointing to lower pain improvement rates with repeat surgeries. The earlier a woman has surgery, the more surgeries she is also likely to have. This is something worth remembering when we consider the push for early diagnosis of endometriosis.

Excision versus ablation

Many women who have endometriosis are of the opinion that excisional surgery (where the endometriosis lesion is carefully dissected off any underlying and surrounding structures and excised completely) is superior to ablation – an older technique where laser or diathermy (heat energy) is used to destroy the endometriosis lesion. As a gynaecological surgeon, I perform excisional surgery because it's safer, more precise and allows for tissue diagnosis of the lesion. But when it comes to pain outcomes, there's no evidence that it's vastly superior to excision. A Cochrane review showed that the effect on pain symptoms was the same whether ablative or excisional surgery was performed for superficial lesions.

Rethinking our approach to endometriosis and pelvic pain

A 2000 letter to the editor of the *British Medical Journal* stated that 'The definitive treatment of endometriosis is simple: surgical eradication' and that 'the success of surgical treatment is best assessed by determining how much disease, if any, remains after operative intervention'. This lesion-focused view of endometriosis and pelvic pain has characterised much of the work on pelvic pain in women over the past few decades. Its entire philosophy of destroying a lesion – which may or may not have anything to do with a woman's pain – misses the point entirely.

CASE STUDY: MARIA AND LUISA

Maria and her mum, Luisa, came to see me because of Maria's painful heavy periods. She was less than a year into menstruating. She had been placed on the Pill to help with her periods after six months, but her periods were still painful. Maria said she initially thought her level of pain was 'normal', but her mum – who has a history of endometriosis – assured her it wasn't.

Maria described a period early on that was so heavy she bled all over her sheets. Her mum wasn't home and she felt terrified. She didn't have pain at the time but she was scared because she'd heard her mum's stories and was expecting history to repeat itself. I'll leave Maria's story here, because the point I want to illustrate about surgery and endometriosis actually belongs to her mum, Luisa.

Luisa told me she'd had painful periods since her first period at 13. She thought her pain was normal until she saw a GP, who referred her to a gynaecologist for a laparoscopy. She was 17 when she had her first laparoscopy, which gave her the diagnosis of endometriosis. This was more than 20 years ago, so Luisa's early diagnosis was ahead of its time and something that many people in the endometriosis community think we should all be aiming for with girls and women who have painful periods. I respectfully disagree.

You might think that if early diagnosis and treatment is gold standard that this early diagnosis and treatment would have set Luisa up for the best chance of a pain-free life. Unfortunately, as for so many other women, surgery was not the magic bullet.

Luisa went on to have five more laparoscopies over the years for ongoing pain, but she was able to conceive all three of her children naturally. She ended up having a hysterectomy for her pain and endometriosis, but this still wasn't the end of it. Sitting in the chair in front of me, she told me that she still had chronic pelvic pain and even had another laparoscopy to remove remaining endometriosis after her hysterectomy – which of course was no more successful at treating her pain.

The point with Luisa's story is that even though she had an early diagnosis, seven surgeries and hormonal suppression – in other words, she was treated in accordance with the standard model of the best care for women with pelvic and period pain – after many years she still had debilitating pelvic pain. How on earth can we continue to believe this biomedical model of treatment is the best care for women with pain?

My job is to do my best to ensure that Maria's life course is very different from her mother's and that she gets the holistic treatment for pain that she needs.

When we zoom out and look at the entire woman, it's clear that surgery and hormonal treatments alone are failing women with pain – whether or not they have endometriosis. Surgery is not a magic bullet for pain, and even if we ascribe most pain to endometriosis (which as we have seen is problematic), surgery does not address any of the upstream causes of endometriosis, such as immune system dysfunction and its possible root causes.

What we are missing is a bio-psycho-social approach, which was an important part of my undergraduate medical degree at a progressive university. But during my gynaecology training, the only thing we were taught about how to help women with pelvic pain was the biomedical, which missed so much of what's important in understanding this pain. As convenient as it would be to find a single cause with a simple surgical cure, my clinical experience and the evidence tells me that we can't pin it all on endometriosis.

The elephant in the room here is that surgery is often not the most effective first-line approach to pelvic pain or endometriosis. It's not a cure; there are less invasive ways of diagnosing endometriosis, such as imaging; and it doesn't reliably fix pain or correct the underlying immune and nervous system factors at play, let alone address any of the other causes of chronic pelvic pain. Dr Mathew Leonardi, a prominent Canadian endometriosis surgeon, recently described surgery in the face of improved imaging as the 'copper standard' for the diagnosis of endometriosis. So why is surgery still held up as the gold standard in the investigation and treatment of chronic pelvic pain in women?

Surgeons, gynaecologists and other stakeholders have the best of intentions, but there are system-wide reasons that maintain this paradigm as the best standard of care. The first of these is that in modern Western medicine, both providers and consumers are invested in the idea of the quick fix, the silver bullet and a pill for every ill. We're all seduced by the promise that surgery will relieve pain. Individual gynaecologists who have found 'something' to see and remove in a woman's pelvis consider their job done if the endometriosis is excised. Surgically it's very satisfying, especially when you've studied and trained for years to gain the technical skills needed to perform safe and complete surgeries. These doctors want to believe that it's helping more than the evidence tells us. I was one of them.

MY STORY: THE INEFFICACY OF SURGERY

To have spent years training and working under the assumption that treating endometriosis by performing surgery helps women with pain, only to come to the conclusion that it's barely scratching the surface and potentially causing more harm than good, is a terribly inconvenient and soul-crushing place to land.

In the early part of my career I did what I was trained to do and offered laparoscopy to exclude or diagnose endometriosis, often without really understanding just what little evidence there was to recommend it. I was like many others who hear 'endometriosis' and think of it as an enemy that must be sought out and crushed. I was trained in that biomedical model where endometriosis – no matter how insignificant – represented disease and was thus the cause of pain.

In my years working in the public system this seemed adequate. The surgery was done and the endometriosis was successfully removed. If they had endometriosis, the patients were most often happy to have a diagnosis and finally feel validated; and when they visited the clinic six weeks later, most felt their pain had lessened. Many times, as it was a public clinic, I wouldn't even be the doctor getting to follow up with the patients post-operatively, so in my short-term view, they were treated and that was that. I was doing my part.

When I entered private practice, with greater continuity of contact with my patients, and more time to explore other possible contributors to pain, I began to realise that the old approach was inadequate. I saw my patients 6 months, then 12 months and then 2 years later when their pain had returned despite the excisional surgery and the prescribing of hormonal medications as I had been trained to do. I'd been trained by, and worked alongside, some of the most highly regarded surgeons in Australia. Why was this happening? Most women, especially those with chronic pain, didn't respond well to conventional endometriosis treatment.

The realisation that the approach I had been taught was often nowhere near enough to successfully address women's suffering was earth-shattering. I wished that it was as simple as we have been led to believe. I wished that I could do an operation and suppress periods and have quick 45-minute initial appointments with women, and that this would fix their pain. But I couldn't and I can't.

I soon knew that I needed to learn more and acquire the necessary tools to help women with pelvic pain more completely.

Many clinicians, even if they recognise the flaws in the current paradigm, haven't learnt about pain from a more holistic viewpoint and lack the skills or time to invest in getting to the root of the problem. The idea that the approach they've been taught might be doing more harm than good for the vast majority of women with pain is confronting, not just because it brings their training into question, but also because it threatens their very livelihood. The medical system itself makes money by doing operations, not by offering multidisciplinary care to women.

When I worked in a public hospital adolescent clinic, I was told that I spent too long talking to my patients, and because the hospital was paid more by the government for procedures than for consultations or allied health referrals, I wasn't meeting my KPIs. Waiting lists for women to see dieticians, psychologists and physiotherapists were sometimes up to a year long, and my requests for allied health staff to work alongside the doctors in my clinic were denied because, while the hospital got paid for surgeries, it would cost money to employ allied health practitioners. The outcome for women wasn't being considered, just the fee for service.

Because of this model, a world in which only 40 per cent of women with persistent pain and endometriosis may benefit from a laparoscopy, not to mention the 30–50 per cent who don't have endometriosis at laparoscopy is very confronting. If we acknowledged the low level of benefit for women, the entire model would need to change. Pelvic pain and endometriosis are often spoken about in terms of their huge financial cost to society. The current paradigm is costing the government hugely in the expense of surgery, even if it's good for the bottom line of the individual hospitals. It's in their financial interests to be doing more surgery, not less.

Gynaecology isn't the only area of medicine where the effectiveness of common surgeries for pain has been questioned. Orthopaedics – a specialty that deals with bones and joints – has been under the spotlight in recent years for procedures such as knee and shoulder arthroscopies, which have been found in clinical trials to be no better than placebo. Other operations such as spinal fusion have shown similar results. MRI imaging often shows meniscal tears and disc and vertebral abnormalities in people who are not experiencing pain. Just as with endometriosis, there is evidence that anatomical changes seen on scans or during a procedure have a poor correlation with pain.

Surgery for superficial endometriosis: helpful or harmful?

So far there is little evidence that shows surgery to treat superficial endometriosis improves pain or quality of life.

Two ongoing high-quality studies are evaluating whether laparoscopic excision for superficial peritoneal endometriosis is helpful or harmful. One, occurring in Denmark, is designed as a double-blinded, randomised controlled trial – the gold-standard design for evidence-based medicine. This particular trial is comparing levels of pelvic pain, general neuroplastic pain symptoms and quality of life across three groups being treated with different interventions: diagnostic laparoscopy with excision of endometriosis, purely diagnostic laparoscopy (sham surgery), or delayed surgery (the no-surgery control group).

The other is a large multicentre trial based in the UK. The investigators note in their summary of why they are doing the research that '80 per cent of women have superficial peritoneal endometriosis (SPE) and many women get limited pain relief from surgical removal of SPE'. Their study design is to randomly assign women to two surgical groups, both undergoing diagnostic laparoscopy, but only one having lesions removed. The aim is 'determining whether surgical removal improves overall symptoms and quality of life or whether surgery is of no benefit, exacerbates symptoms or even causes harm'.

I eagerly anticipate the results of these studies, so that I can provide women and caregivers with actual data about the perceived benefits of surgery or lack thereof. Until then we have to be mindful that there is currently insufficient good-quality evidence for the effectiveness of surgery.

Experts, special interest groups and endometriosis sufferers wrote the first *Endometriosis Clinical Practice Guideline* for Australia in 2021. These guidelines say it all about the level of evidence when it comes to endometriosis and more importantly pelvic pain. Almost all its recommendations are made based on very low to low levels of evidence, which means that further research is very likely to change our approach to diagnosis and surgical management. There is much research to be done into the cause of and best treatment for women's pain.

Surgery is not necessary to validate a woman's pain

Women want to be heard. Often the first time they feel heard or their pain is taken seriously is when a caring and well-meaning doctor says, 'Your pain is not normal. It might be endometriosis and there's an operation for that.' It might not even be a doctor telling them that these days. It might be another young woman, telling her own story using a platform such as TikTok, YouTube or Instagram. There are also many advocacy and peer support groups built around helping women with endometriosis connect. While anything that helps to build connection in an increasingly disconnected world is a good thing, many of these groups treat endometriosis as an identity. Women understandably feel like they've had to fight for their lives to get their pain heard and validated so it's not surprising that many wear their laparoscopy incision sites like battle scars and call themselves 'endo warriors'.

But what of the many women who have pelvic pain but don't have endometriosis? The urge to belong to a group with a 'biological' cause for pain is strong, particularly a disease with the cachet of endometriosis because our purely pelvic-centred medical model only validates women who have a diagnosis of endometriosis. I have seen countless women throughout my career burst into tears in the recovery room after a laparoscopy has failed to identify endometriosis. Where is their place? Without the diagnosis of endometriosis, they do not get validation for their pain. The current medical model doesn't have much to offer them, and because of the limited understanding of the complexity of pain in the wider community, they often feel unsupported, alone and, worst of all, like the pain is all in their head.

Except it's not. It permeates their being and has just as devastating an effect on their quality of life as does pain in women who also happen to have endometriosis. Even for those women who have pain and a diagnosis of endometriosis, their pain may be caused by something other than endometriosis.

If there is more to it than endometriosis, if the solution is more complex than surgery or a drug, then in many ways it's incredibly disheartening. It would mean an overhaul in the way we treat women with pain. For a start it would mean listening to and validating women's pain *all* of the time. It would mean that doctors allocate more time to listening to women's stories and getting to the root of the problem by considering not just the biological but also the psychological and social, and the ways these factors can affect the biological.

It would mean that the healthcare system starts to put in place an outcome-based rather than procedure-based model, providing financial incentives for the holistic and multidisciplinary care women need for pelvic pain. It would mean that gynaecologists move on from focusing on lesions to looking at the whole woman, which could mean less surgery and more upskilling in treating pain. It would mean doing the work of addressing the root causes of chronic pelvic pain, which for many women can be confronting, especially as support is lacking. At a societal level, it would mean facing the complexity of issues leading to the development of chronic pain – including childhood trauma, sexism, and the mismatch between female biology and the pace and expectations of capitalist modern life.

I am hopeful that things are starting to change. Other gynaecologists and doctors who work with women experiencing pelvic pain understand that biological reductionism at the expense of the psycho-social is not serving women. The recent Australian *Endometriosis Clinical Practice Guideline* stated that treatment for endometriosis should be offered 'according to the person's symptoms, preferences and priorities rather than the stage of endometriosis' and that treatment should be 'patient-focused, considering the person's physical, psychological, sexual, social, spiritual and cultural needs and preferences'.

I wholeheartedly agree with this – except that I would replace 'endometriosis' with 'pelvic pain'. This is not a book about endometriosis. This is a book about everything that contributes to the development of chronic pelvic pain. In most cases they are related to the effects of a sick society rather than inherently flawed and broken women.

Chapter summary

- The true effect of surgery in improving pelvic pain is around 40 per cent, taking into account a 30 per cent placebo effect (improvement in women who had surgery incisions but no treatment).
- Up to half of the women who improve will have a recurrence of pain and go on to have a repeat surgery within 5 years.
- 30–50 per cent of women undergoing laparoscopy for pain will not have endometriosis.
- Women most likely to benefit from surgery are those with cyclical pain or deep lesions.
- Women least likely to benefit from surgery are those with pain on most days or women who are having repeat surgery.
- Surgery will never address the huge influence of the nervous system, the gut and immune system on chronic pain.

6

Moving beyond the biomedical model

Fortunately, there is now increasing awareness of pelvic pain and especially endometriosis in women. Unfortunately, the focus is still mainly on endometriosis lesions and surgery, while the other extremely important factors involved in pelvic pain often get left out of the conversation entirely. As a result, many women continue to have pain despite surgery, while many others are left feeling lost and invalidated if their surgery did not reveal endometriosis and yet they still experience pain.

I am passionate about opening up this very narrow view on pelvic pain and shining the spotlight on the other factors that drive pain. Modern medicine has landed firmly on the biomedical perspective, but this isn't working and it's failing women. To truly hear and address each individual woman's pain at the root, it's imperative to explore the specific psychological and social factors at play. There are buckets of evidence not only that these massive parts of a woman's life contribute to the experience of physical pain, but also that they have a very real physical effect on the body which, as we will see in the next chapter, can increase the likelihood of pain.

The West's separation of mind and body

We live in dualistic society that separates us from one other, from nature and from the world around us – even from parts of ourselves. During the conceptualisation of Western medicine, the idea of mind–body dualism formed the basis of the biomedical model through which we view health and disease today. Mind–body dualism is the philosophy that the mind and body are completely separate entities. René Descartes, the 17th-century philosopher most famous for writing 'I think therefore I am', made this school of thought a cornerstone of the Enlightenment.

Separating the mind, spirit or soul from the physical body at this time paved the way for tearing medicine away from religious dogma and towards the scientific study of anatomy, biology and physiology. It began the process of mechanising the physical body, breaking it down into parts to be studied, and resulted in the biological reductionism that meant only what could be seen was real. Disease began to be viewed as a deviation from biological norms and caused by physical or chemical changes. (Obviously this is a problem when it comes to women's health, because even today we're yet to determine exactly what is normal in the female body.) The cure for disease was then the introduction of a physical (surgical) or chemical (pharmaceutical) agent to bring the body back into a state of biological normality.

Both the medical profession and women suffering from pain help to uphold this mind–body dualism. Most practitioners aren't even aware that they're practising within this philosophical framework – it has become an embedded way of thinking. We see this so often, when something doesn't fit into this model it is treated as 'not real'. Any other explanation that tries to bring in the psycho-social is often seen as nonsense or imaginary. The idea of something only being 'real' if it fulfils the biological–physical criteria is so pervasive that it affects how women with pain are treated by doctors and leads those women on a quest for the biological cause of their pain.

Women want to be validated, and their conditioning has taught them that if they don't fit this model they won't be validated, heard or treated. Sometimes even in my own practice, when I begin to ask women about their psychological state or their social situation or a past history of trauma, many think that by making a connection between their emotions and their physical pain I am being dismissive. All they can hear is that their pain is not real, that they are crazy and making it up.

Mind–body dualism and pelvic pain

When we become aware of the soup we're swimming in, it makes total sense why doctors seek to find and treat lesions and why women are so desperate to have a biological cause found and treated. They fear falling outside the biomedical model and being lost in a wilderness that doesn't see or treat their pain. I think this is why women with pelvic pain have so embraced endometriosis as *the* cause for their pain, and why some identify as 'endo warriors'.

For the first time, their pain and their experiences are legitimised. They are not crazy, it's not their fault. The hope and optimism that come with the promise of a simple surgical fix for their pain is tantalising. For many women, it also means they now belong to a group. When we're suffering from pain, our sense of connection to self and also others is often poor, but to belong to a group of women for whom a powerful authority figure has confirmed 'Your pain is real' feels validating on so many levels.

The greater the medical authority deems the severity of their endometriosis, the more validated they feel. To have stage 4 endometriosis gives you more cachet than mild or grade 1 disease. The trouble is, there's rarely ever a correlation between extent of disease and severity of symptoms, which is one of the main arguments against endometriosis being the main driver of pelvic pain. The medical field and society as a whole have been slow to accept the notion that there are other reasons for pain that don't fit neatly into the surgical model of disease.

Resistance to change

When the Australian endometriosis guidelines were published in 2021, there was huge backlash from people in the 'endometriosis community' over surgical excision not being promoted as the gold standard of treatment. As we have seen, there is currently no evidence that excision is any better for pain than ablation. It may be tempting to believe, if you've had ablation surgery but are still in pain, that excisional surgery, particularly for superficial endometriosis, will be the answer, but the science simply doesn't bear this out. The other factor in the excision versus ablation debate is that most women who undergo ablation have mild disease, whereas excisional surgery is always needed if a deep lesion is to be removed. Mild endometriosis is probably the least likely to respond to surgical treatment of any kind because it may not even be the main cause of the woman's pain.

The guidelines also promoted a holistic approach to treating pain and endometriosis, with or without surgery, based on what was important to each individual patient. This could include treatments such as hormones and physiotherapy for pain. It speaks volumes that these guidelines were partly written by doctors who are experts in endometriosis and who perform surgical excision of endometriosis for a living. To consider a conservative approach and to acknowledge that there's not enough evidence to always recommend surgery for pain demonstrates that even doctors with a vested interest in surgery can see that biological reductionism is not working for women with pelvic pain.

Women with endometriosis who disapproved of the guidelines believed that without surgery their endometriosis would continue to grow. They felt that they were almost being gaslit into treating pain rather than endometriosis. We have already seen that most endometriosis is stable or regresses – but this position highlights the misinformation that exists at a community-wide level.

They launched a petition calling for more excisional surgery centres, and diagnostic and therapeutic laparoscopies for everyone with pain so as not to 'miss endometriosis'. But we know that endometriosis is not always the cause of pain and that mild endometriosis may not even represent a disease state. We also know that modern pain science tells us that persistent pain is unlikely to be helped with surgery. Despite this, these massive social media accounts continue to feed young women misinformation, fuelling fear which, when you understand the neurobiology of pain, is contributing to pain.

Mind *and* matter

We know instinctively that the mind and our experiences in the world can affect our physical health. We need only look at the growing popularity in the West of mind–body therapies and non-dualistic traditional health philosophies – such as Ayurveda, Chinese medicine and South American shamanism. Many women do seek alternative therapies for their endometriosis and/or pelvic pain when the traditional Western approach has failed.

As far back as 1947, the World Health Organization's Constitution stated that 'Health is a state of complete physical, mental and social well-being, and not merely the absence of disease or infirmity.' In the 1990s, US doctor and holistic treatment advocate Alvin Tarlov expanded upon this, defining health as 'the capacity, relative to potential and aspirations, for living fully in the social environment'.

This is why, at my progressive university during my undergraduate degree, the biomedical approach was thrown out in favour of the bio-psycho-social model. While medicine has adopted this approach for many other conditions, for women with pelvic pain we're still firmly stuck in the dualistic way of thinking.

I recall an emergency physician calling me when one of my patients was being admitted with a pelvic pain flare. When I discussed her care plan, which involved talking to her, reinforcing the effect on her pain of her current emotional state, employing positive self-talk and pelvic relaxation, he said, 'Why do you always get these types of women? It's like you practise a kind of gynae-psychiatry.' This comment epitomises mind–body dualism in medicine. Being a gynaecologist involves more than just treating a woman as a uterus with ovaries and a vagina. It involves treating a whole woman, whose emotions, experiences and nervous system are involved in symptoms that may appear purely gynaecological at first. In my view, our parts cannot be broken down into separate entities. If I am treating a woman, I treat all of her.

The mind–body bridge: the nervous system

Human beings are dynamic creatures, constantly responding to their environment in physical and emotional ways. In this sense we can't be separated into mind and body – there is a continuum; we are one and the same. Our mind and body, just as they can't be separated from one another, can't be separated from our environment – including our immediate environment and the wider cultural soup we swim in. The bridge between our body and our mind is our nervous system, which responds to danger in our environment and induces changes in our body that can alter our biology – right down to the cellular level.

Explaining this bridge is the key to helping women understand that we don't need to diagnose endometriosis for their pain to be real. Pain is always real, whether or not we find physical evidence during a laparoscopy. Validation of a woman's pain experience should not come after an operation, but right at the start, simply by listening to her whole story. By accepting a woman's pain story at face value, then exploring her history by looking at not only the physical but also her childhood, the dynamics around her as she was growing up, prevailing views to menstruation, and her social and psychological state, we can start to build a picture that can almost always identify and explain all the specific factors at play in the development of her individual pelvic pain.

Whether or not you *might* have endometriosis is almost irrelevant. It's far more likely that other factors are driving your pain. The diagnosis of endometriosis isn't the issue. It's the years of ignoring women and failing to identify all the factors that may be part of her story. This is where we need to start. When I talk to women about pain, whether or not they have a diagnosis of endometriosis, we can often identify several big players. It's hardly ever just endometriosis. Failing to identify these other drivers of pain may be part of the reason why surgical and hormonal treatments for endometriosis are often not enough to treat pain, and why women are going back for more and more surgeries. With women who don't have endometriosis, failing to address these other incredibly important factors leaves them in the wilderness of 'all in your head' and left outside the endometriosis community.

If you have pelvic pain and you feel lost as to its drivers, or if your doctor is only offering endometriosis as a cause and your treatment is focused purely on eradicating lesions – then it is imperative that you know there are other answers. This book will help you identify what may be driving pain in your unique body. When you understand these causes and effects, you will not only have less fear about what's happening in your body, but you will have the power to address them. The key is to bring the mind and body together as one – what affects one, affects the other.

The importance of recognising trauma

In my practice, more than 90 per cent of women I see with persistent pelvic pain have experienced significant developmental trauma and/or are experiencing high ongoing stress. In my view, the way that trauma (particularly in childhood or adolescence) or ongoing high perceived stress impacts the body at a physical level affects our likelihood of experiencing pain. For many people this idea feels dismissive, which is understandable if they consider the biomedical model to be superior to the bio-psycho-social model.

But more and more scientific evidence supports the fact that what we feel and what we think changes our physicality. When we feel scared, stressed or angry, we release stress hormones that have direct effects on our physiology in almost every system of our body. Our mind and body have never been separate entities, and when we refuse to acknowledge the mental, emotional, environmental, social and cultural factors that influence our biology, our understanding of what constitutes real health remains incomplete and we're unable to develop effective treatments. We already know that stress and microbiome disruption can result in leaky gut and immune changes that upregulate inflammation in the nervous system through TLR 4 cells, which bridge the immune and nervous systems. The concept of everything being connected is called psychoneuroimmunology and basically explains the mind-body continuum.

I believe that when we can explain the effects of trauma on our biology, we can finally see the mind–body–environment continuum as a whole *and* explain pain and other physical effects of trauma. Science has illustrated the ways stress and trauma affect our bodies. There is no longer any need for a dismissive 'It's all in your head'. The effects of trauma and stress are as real as a spot of endometriosis found in your pelvis by your surgeon – but they might explain your pain more completely.

It's incredibly confronting to think that your pain may have something to do with your nervous system's response to previous trauma or ongoing stress – both from the point of view of your own suffering and the medical system. Dealing with trauma and stress requires much more time and work than a quick consultation and an operation. From the bigger-picture view, it requires society-wide changes to look at and address the epidemic of childhood trauma and the way we often dismiss and add to the stress of women in our culture. This might not be your story. But there's a good chance it is – especially if the conventional treatment for endometriosis hasn't worked or you don't have endometriosis but continue to suffer with pain.

We are not simple creatures and our pain cannot be addressed simply by cutting bits of ourselves away or turning off the hormonal cycles that make us women. We are complex, whole and exist within a system that affects our experience in the world. To get to the root of the matter, we must accept that these factors are just as real and important. We must learn to listen to the language of pain. What is your pain trying to tell you? Although it may sound counterintuitive, when we surrender and embrace our pain, we are able to listen to its message. When we try at any cost to quash pain, deny it and wish it away, then it screams ever louder to get our attention.

Modern pain science tells us that the majority of people suffering chronic pain have neuroplastic pain – pain generated by the brain. For most women with chronic pain, who also happen to have been diagnosed with endometriosis, this is also true. Failing to recognise or treat pain with the complexity it deserves sells women incredibly short, and ends up damaging more women than it helps. Denying the relevance of the mind–body connection means that women with persistent pain are receiving substandard treatment that is not up to date with our current understanding of pain science.

CASE STUDY: LUCY

Lucy was 27 when she came to see me. On her intake form she wrote of feeling as though endometriosis had taken everything from her. She attributed the pain she began feeling immediately upon the onset of her periods at 14 to her endometriosis, which went on to be diagnosed via a laparoscopy at the age of 20. Her pain decreased a little after her first surgery but soon came back, and she ended up having another laparoscopy at 25, which showed only old scar tissue and no active endometriosis.

Lucy had a Mirena IUD and, although she had occasional light bleeding, did not have periods any more. Despite this, her pain persisted and was now there almost all the time. Lucy wrote on her intake form: 'My endo rules my life. It controls what I eat, what I do throughout the day and my anxiety. I have PTSD [post-traumatic stress disorder] with everyday activities because I am worried about how they might activate my endo.'

She also wrote that despite her belief that her pain was due to her endometriosis, she first started having pelvic pain when she was 10. Lucy disclosed that at this time in her life she was sexually abused by her stepfather for a period of two years. She said, 'I didn't have endometriosis at this point, just horrible pain from the sexual abuse.'

Lucy's emotionally immature mother hadn't believed her when she finally disclosed her abuse at the age of 16. When writing about her relationship with her mother as a child she said, 'My mother wasn't very supportive and to be honest, she was someone who shouldn't have kids. I was an angry child and did naughty things all the time.' This indicates a constant feeling of not being safe in her environment or with the people who were supposed to protect her. She also stated that she suffered from severe depression for most of her teenage years. She tried to commit suicide at 16, and her relationship with her mother continued to be both physically and emotionally abusive.

Lucy was now training as an officer in the army, but felt like her endometriosis was a barrier to achieving career success because it reinforced the 'weak woman with period issues' stereotype. She strove to push it and anything relating to her femininity away, as the only way she felt she could achieve her goals was to deny her own biology and behave like a man. Lucy said that as bad as endometriosis was for her life and career, at least it gave her a legitimacy, with a valid biologically based disease.

She struggled with body image, bloating and gastro-intestinal issues. While she had a supportive long-term partner, she was unable to have sex without pain. She had been seeing a pelvic floor physiotherapist to help with relaxing her pelvic muscles, but she maintained the issue wasn't her muscles but her 'angry uterus and cervix'. She believed that sex was excruciating when her cervix was touched, and this fed into her narrative that if only her uterus and cervix could be removed, she might be able to live a normal, pain-free life again.

While Lucy was also seeing a psychologist to address her anxiety, self-esteem issues and painful sex, she did not feel able to talk to anyone in her life about what had happened to her when she was 10 years old. After being shut down and disbelieved by her mother, Lucy understandably became very reluctant to tell anyone else, for fear of being shamed or not believed. This ongoing sense of not feeling safe was compounded by her choice to pursue a career in the army, where a history of trauma and mental health issues is actively frowned upon.

When we talked about her history of sexual abuse and the complex PTSD she likely had as a result of growing up feeling unsafe, she recognised that this was where her pain started and not with endometriosis or her periods. She could see that the consequences of her body trying to keep her safe at a time when she was not safe had activated parts of her nervous system that made her hypervigilant to anything that could be perceived as a danger signal. Painful stimuli became more painful, and sometimes sensations that most people wouldn't perceive as painful, became so – all because her brain was misinterpreting a safe signal as a danger signal because of fear. Lucy could understand this and knew that a lot of her trauma was unprocessed and was consequently having an impact on her physical body.

Because Lucy was primed to experience pain right back in childhood, when the volume dial on her nervous system was turned way up high, her periods were likely more painful than they would have been otherwise. Because of her pain, her doctors went looking for endometriosis, which they found. Lucy admitted to me how compelling the idea was that her pain was caused by a collection of cells that could be removed, and how it enabled her to finally experience a degree of recognition and compassion for her suffering. It gave her pain a validity she hadn't felt before. It gave her hope that by excising the 'broken' parts of her body and turning off the hormones that reminded her of the existence of her uterus, her pain would go away.

But despite surgery and hormones that took away periods, her pain increased until it was constant and daily. The fact that her second laparoscopy failed to show any further endometriosis is evidence that it was likely not her endometriosis causing her ongoing pain. I would even argue that it may not have been the driver of her pain in the first place.

Lucy told me that neither of her previous two gynaecologists or her GPs had ever asked about her childhood or adolescence, or her history of anxiety, depression and sexual trauma. This was the first time she felt she could tell her story. Without an operation, without changing any medications, she felt validated. She began to realise that maybe her body wasn't broken. Maybe it had been trying to protect her all this time.

After we spoke for more than an hour, Lucy felt safe enough to have an examination to explore what she 'knew to be true' about the sensations in her body. Lucy had overactive and tight pelvic floor muscles, but when I touched her cervix – which she had said was incredibly sensitive and was the cause of pain when she had sex – she felt no sensation. We did an ultrasound and I could tell her that her uterus and ovaries looked normal and beautiful; she felt no pain with the examination.

She had previously been diagnosed with an ovarian cyst – but to me it sounded like it was an ovarian follicle, a normal part of the ovaries working to release an egg each month. I showed her that she had another follicle on one of her ovaries but it had no concerning features and was a sign that her ovaries were doing exactly what they are supposed to do. I used positive and empowering language with Lucy to describe the parts of her that had been blamed as the sole reason for her pain.

When I could teach Lucy that her cervix and her uterus weren't the cause of her pain, she could begin to experience safety in her body and start to challenge some of her beliefs about the cause of her pain. I saw her only a few months later and she had been able to settle any pain flares by reminding herself that she was safe and that no tissue damage was occurring.

While endometriosis might be part of the story, it is rarely the whole story, and by focusing on it exclusively it's as if we're removing the tip of an iceberg – only to leave the rest lurking beneath the surface of the water unseen. Those suffering with pelvic pain deserve better.

Chapter summary

- Western medicine has evolved to separate the mind and the body, which reduces pain to a 'structural' cause.
- If no structural cause is found, women feel that their pain must all be in their head.
- There is a validation that comes from the medical community for a 'physical' cause but not from a cause rooted in the nervous system.
- Misinformation in the online space about endometriosis continues to drive fear and push women towards seeking treatments like surgery that alone are unlikely to be effective for persistent pain.

7

Understanding pain

As you can now see, having visible endometriosis lesions does not necessarily produce pain or chronic pelvic pain. We have to cast the net wider and look deeper into the nervous system for answers.

At the most basic level, most of us understand that pain is an unpleasant sensation that is usually caused by actual or potential tissue damage. Pain is also subjective – in that everyone's sensation of pain is different and influenced by biological, psychological, social and cultural factors.

Different types of pain

There are various types of pain, but they include nociceptive pain, neuropathic pain and neuroplastic pain (pain system hypersensitivity). Many women with chronic pelvic pain have both nociceptive and neuroplastic pain.

Nociceptive pain

Nociceptive or acute pain is a way for our brain to recognise and respond to danger in our environment so as to avoid or minimise tissue damage. It's the kind of pain we might have with inflammation from an infection or injury. Period pain due to inflammatory chemicals released by the uterus lining to allow it to shed is also an example of this kind of pain – although when severe or chronic it can become more complicated than this. The most important thing to remember though is that most of the time the pain that comes with periods is not causing tissue damage and is usually not dangerous.

Nociceptive pain can be somatic or visceral. Somatic pain comes from muscles, bones and soft tissues while visceral pain comes from internal organs. Often women with pelvic pain may have both types of pain; somatic from tense muscles in the pelvic floor and visceral from inflammation around the pelvic organs, such as the uterus, bladder and bowel, due to periods and/or endometriosis.

Acute pain is a vital survival mechanism for keeping us safe. When our nervous system is working correctly, dangerous stimuli are converted into a pain signal by the brain and we can get the help we need. In this sort of situation, pain is a protective response that conveys an evolutionary advantage to help us survive. But the activation of nociceptors doesn't always produce pain – the brain decides whether to activate a pain response based on bio-psyche-social factors and in the context of previous experiences. This is what makes the sensation of acute pain highly individual.

We're taught to think that if we have pelvic pain it's always because of something dangerous happening in the pelvis. There are of course structural or anatomical conditions that do cause acute pain, and these need to be ruled out or treated in an urgent time frame. For example, if pain is due to appendicitis, a ruptured ectopic pregnancy or something dangerous, the brain is interpreting danger signals from peripheral nerves in the pelvis correctly and producing pain to alert you that you need attention. These kinds of pain usually don't wax and wane and generally get worse. They are diagnosable with ultrasound, CT scan or blood tests, and can be assessed and treated by a GP or emergency department. Once the cause is treated and the danger has passed, the pain usually goes away. This is an adaptive form of pain that helps us survive.

But with persistent period or pelvic pain the usual causes are less sinister:

- inflammation from prostaglandins released as part of the shedding of the uterus lining
- endometrial cells or blood coming back into the pelvis and irritating the pelvis lining (retrograde menstruation, a normal part of getting your period)
- inflammation from endometriosis sensitising other organs in the pelvis such as the bowel or bladder or pelvic floor
- pelvic floor muscle tension
- constipation, bloating and/or gut pain
- upregulated pain pathways – pain system hypersensitivity.

Neuropathic pain

Nerve pain or neuropathic pain generally results from damage to peripheral nerves, the pain or touch nerves that transfer sensory information from the brain and spinal cord to other parts of the body. Neuropathic pain can occur as a result of nerve injury during surgery, an accident or childbirth. It often feels like a burning, shooting or electric-shock sensation that occurs without provocation. It can also feel like pins and needles or numbness.

Neuroplastic pain – pain system hypersensitivity

The most common cause of chronic or persistent pain, brain-generated or neuroplastic pain, is far more complex, because the legitimate and often severe pain we feel is usually not due to tissue damage or a real danger. Neuroplastic pain simply refers to changes in the nervous system that result in amplification of the pain signal transmitted to the brain and the misinterpretation of safe sensations as dangerous ones.

Chronic pain is usually defined as pain that occurs on most days for greater than three months. Acute pain resulting from an injury, surgery or an acute condition can transform into chronic pelvic pain, but often for women it occurs over time without an obvious trigger at first. Particularly painful periods that remain unmanaged are commonly associated with the development of chronic pelvic pain – either in the context of a diagnosis of endometriosis or not. As we saw from Chapter 3, the same molecular and cellular processes can occur in women with pelvic pain regardless of the cause. For example, endometriosis, infection and even just painful periods cause the immune cells TLR4 to turn up pain pathways in the central nervous system. This is why prompt treatment of ongoing debilitating period pain is so important to reduce the risk of developing chronic pain. Chronic pelvic pain can also occur after pregnancy or childbirth. And you will see later in this book, many of the women who see me have histories of sexual trauma or other traumas that preceded their development of pelvic pain.

Pain system hypersensitivity is not due to ongoing danger or tissue damage but results from a faulty pain pathway system. To understand persistent pelvic pain in women with or without endometriosis, we need to take a look at the body's entire pain perception system. Not understanding the complexity of chronic pelvic pain, and simplistically judging all pain to be caused by something dangerous in the pelvis, frequently perpetuates that pain because it keeps us stuck in old models of treatment that aren't working. Doing 10 laparoscopies to remove endometriosis as a therapy for pain is ineffective because it neglects the parts of the pain pathway system that are most likely causing the majority of the ongoing pain. And all too often it makes pain worse by adding injury, painful stimuli and further scar tissue.

How the brain perceives pain

Our nervous system is like a complex network of highways, roads and pathways that sends messages from our brain to all over our body and from our body through sensation back to the brain. It comprises the central nervous system (our brain and spinal cord) and the peripheral nervous system (our touch and pain receptors). But our brain ultimately decides what sensory input is dangerous by constructing a pain sensation. Sometimes it judges correctly and pain is a helpful response, but other times, as is often the case in chronic pain, the brain misinterprets safe sensations as dangerous and so produces a pain response in the absence of tissue damage or legitimate danger.

Pain is contextual and can be upregulated by fear and anxiety. Leading Australian neuroscientist, Dr Lorimer Mosely, in one of his famous TED talks gives a great personal example. Walking through the Australian bush one beautiful day with a good friend, chatting, relaxed and happy, he feels a scratch sensation on his leg and disregards it, until a few minutes later he realises he's been bitten by a snake. He recovers and a year later, in a bid to confront his fears, returns to the same bushwalk. Understandably on both a conscious and subconscious level his nervous system is on high alert, finely attuned to every little bit of incoming sensory information. All of a sudden he feels a searing, burning pain in his foot and is certain he's been bitten again by another snake, but this time he turns and sees that it was just a stick. In this example you can see how Dr Mosely's nervous system, in a fear state, had turned up the volume on every incoming pain signal, which then amplified the innocuous pain of a scratch from a stick. Context is everything.

Pain is an integration of the sensory input coming from the body via the neural pathway (bottom-up signals), and our beliefs, emotions and expectations about the sensation coming from the primitive parts of our brain such as the amygdala and the limbic system (top-down signals). Any fear around the stimulus will increase the sensation of pain because the more fear there is, the more likely the brain will be to perceive the stimulus as dangerous and produce more pain. This is why pain is subjective and two people won't respond with the same level of pain to the same stimulus. The brain also often creates a shortcut called predictive coding, producing a sensation based on what it expects from beliefs and previous experiences rather than an actual stimulus in the body. This can sometimes lead to errors and produce a pain sensation based on a previous painful event when there's no real danger. An example of this is an amputee who has phantom limb pain. The pain is very real but there is no arm or leg to cause the pain. The pain is entirely in the nervous system.

Pain responses to similar stimuli within the same person can also be different at different points in time, depending on other factors that affect the state of the nervous system.

We know that pain is worse when a person is tired, anxious, depressed or suffering a negative emotional state. Science tells us that when we experience emotional pain, the same parts of our brain are activated as when we experience physical pain. One study showed that the somatosensory cortex, the part of the brain associated with physical pain, also lights up when we feel emotional pain from social rejection or by viewing images of a former partner when the break-up is recent and raw.

Sleep deprivation is also associated with an increase in pain. One study evaluated levels of pain in healthy adults, firstly after eight hours' sleep and secondly after they had been kept awake for 24–48 hours. Functional MRI images showed that the sleep-deprived participants had a much lower pain threshold and that the part of their brain involved in pain processing was 120 per cent more active. Researchers also measured a 60–90 per cent decrease in the activity of two areas of the brain that usually inhibit pain perception. Sleep deprivation also increases production of cortisol (our stress hormone) and is known to be associated with higher levels of inflammation, which may have contributed to these changes in pain perception.

Pain system hypersensitivity

A big part of what happens with neuroplastic pain is how it causes pain system hypersensitivity – the term used to explain the way our bottom-up pain pathways become so highly sensitive that the brain begins to interpret not only mildly painful sensations as super painful, but also non-painful stimuli such as touch as painful. This often occurs in conditions such as vulval pain syndromes, where even a light touch with a cotton bud produces exquisite pain. It is also seen with periods, making normal mild period pain feel severe – not because of dangerous tissue damage in the pelvis but because the volume dial on the pain pathway system is turned up to extra loud.

As the diagram on the following page illustrates, when our body's pain-sensing system is operating normally, painful stimuli activate our nociceptors (pain nerves) to produce a pain sensation, while non-painful stimuli activate our touch receptors to produce a safe touch sensation in the brain.

When the nervous system becomes 'sensitised', everything causes a pain sensation, regardless of the stimulus. As the top diagram demonstrates, painful stimuli produce even more intense pain sensations, known as hyperalgesia (literally higher pain), while harmless touch stimuli activate the pain pathways to produce a pain sensation in the absence of any tissue damage or danger, known as allodynia.

Neuroplastic pain is almost always associated at some level with persistent pain. Even if pain started due to endometriosis or actual tissue damage, when it becomes chronic, the nervous system is almost always playing a huge part in perpetuating pain. In fact, in a recent study, almost 80 per cent of women presenting with pelvic pain showed evidence of neuroplastic pain or central sensitisation. In other words, if you have persistent pain, even if you've been diagnosed with endometriosis and feel like all your pain is due to those endometriosis cells, your nervous system is a big part of the driver – and by ignoring it you'll remain stuck in your pain. Women who have persistent pain are probably the least likely to benefit from surgery, because surgery leaves out the nervous system, which is the biggest ongoing driver of chronic pain.

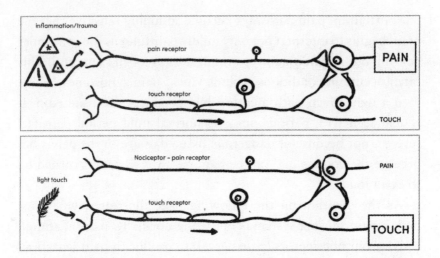

Normal sensitisation

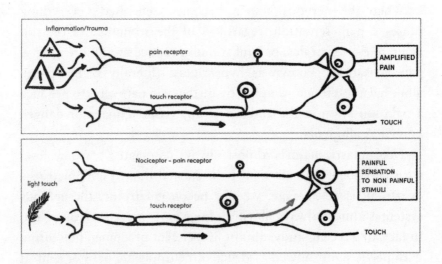

Pain system hypersensitivity

Adapted from CJ Woolf, 'Central sensitization: implications for the diagnosis and treatment of pain', *Pain*, 2011, vol. 152, supplement, pp. S2–S15.

People whose acute pain becomes chronic pain are more likely to have experienced trauma or ongoing stress or have perfectionistic personalities. Research also tells us that fear of the pain or symptom is often an ongoing driver of pain.

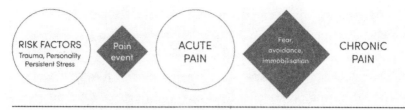

RISK FACTORS
Trauma, Personality
Persistent Stress

Pain event

ACUTE PAIN

Fear, avoidance, immobilisation

CHRONIC PAIN

TIME

Development of chronic pain

MY STORY: HOW MY ACUTE TOOTH PAIN BECAME CHRONIC PAIN

As an example of how neuroplastic or persistent pain works, I often tell my patients about an experience I had with pain. I developed acute pain in my upper back molar that intensified over a few days and was really severe to the point that I couldn't sleep. My dentist diagnosed a fracture that had become infected. This was an example of acute or nociceptive pain – caused by a noxious stimulus: the fracture and the infection.

For context, I often have high anxiety and am a tooth grinder at night. Having had bulimia in my early twenties, I had always feared the dentist and felt a deep shame about how I treated my body at that time in my life. My fear and shame about anything relating to my teeth was huge. No one loves going to the dentist, but I was absolutely petrified at the best of times. To be told I needed root canal therapy dredged up all those feelings of guilt and shame, let alone fear of the pain.

The endodontist told me that because the fracture had extended right down to the root of the tooth, he couldn't go ahead with root canal and the tooth couldn't be saved. I had to have an extraction in the chair, which was one of the worst experiences of my life. After the extraction, the dentist told me to watch out for dry socket, a condition where the gum bed can become infected because the blood clot that was supposed to form falls off, which can cause intense pain. I'd had this when I had a wisdom tooth out many years earlier, so I knew the pain. I also knew to be afraid of it.

Of course, three days later I was convinced that I'd developed this condition because the pain was getting worse again. I went back to see the dentist, who told me all was well and there were no signs of infection. I felt reassured and the pain decreased and went away – coinciding with a beautiful holiday to Fiji with my family where I was relaxed and happy.

About a month later, when I was back at work and under a lot more stress, I started noticing a funny tingling sensation around several of my teeth and then the pain started again. This pain was just like before with the fractured tooth. It was severe, radiating to my jaw, neck and head. At first it started around one tooth and then it moved to involve several. The familiar fear and anxiety started to creep back in. I couldn't sleep. I was preoccupied with the pain, and the thought that all my teeth would need to be pulled out terrified me. My brain was on high alert for danger and interpreted any sensation from my mouth as dangerous.

I called the dentist in a panic and he was able to fit me in the same day. He checked all my teeth meticulously, unable to bring on any sensitivity or pain, and then sat me back up in the chair. He told me with trepidation that there was nothing wrong, that perhaps I needed to see my GP about my anxiety, and gave me a card for a head and neck physiotherapist to treat the tension in my jaw.

I think he was worried I was going to be upset when he gently suggested it was all in my head, but as someone who deals with neuroplastic pain every day and knows it's treatable and definitely preferable to having teeth pulled out, I was relieved. But at the same time I was fascinated that I was experiencing some of the same things my patients go through with their pelvic pain.

Let's summarise what we have learnt so far about the science behind chronic pain:

1. Women potentially experience nociceptive pain each month with periods – but if this is severe, due to increased inflammation or a heightened state of fear, persistent or neuroplastic pain is more likely.
2. The brain learns chronic pain, and fear is important as an ongoing driver of pain.
3. Persistent pain is also associated with activation of TLR4 cells that amplify pain by increasing inflammation in the brain and nervous system.
4. Pain system hypersensitivity – the process of harmless stimuli activating pain pathways – develops when this cycle starts.
5. Pain production is based on a combination of bottom-up processes (pain pathways and stimuli like periods and inflammation) and top-down processes (past experience, emotions, stress, sleep).
6. Emotional pain activates the same part of the brain as physical pain.
7. The longer pain persists untreated, the deeper these neural pathways are carved.
8. Neuroplasticity means that while chronic pain can be learned, it can also be unlearned, which is great news if you have pain.

CASE STUDY: MIRANDA

Miranda was 13 when she first came to see me with her mum. She had been referred to me by another gynaecologist after she had already had surgery for endometriosis. Miranda got her first period at 12 and her periods were painful from the beginning. She was commenced on the oral contraceptive Pill by her GP after only a couple of periods, but although this stopped her periods, it did not improve her pain. Her mood worsened, either because of the effects of pain on her life or as a side effect of the Pill.

Before surgery, Miranda's daily pain was having a huge effect on her quality of life. While she normally loved school, was a studious young woman and a bit of a perfectionist, she was starting to miss more days of school and was unable to participate in the sports she loved. During her laparoscopy, she was found to have superficial widespread endometriosis, mainly on the ligaments that hold up the uterus and in the area between the uterus and the bowel. This was all excised completely by a very competent surgeon.

Unfortunately, while Miranda reported perhaps a brief mild improvement in pain following surgery, her pain soon became even worse than before. She was referred to me because her gynaecologist knew I had an interest in persistent pain. Apart from starting on the Pill, Miranda had no treatment for her persistent pain before surgery.

When I first saw Miranda six months or so after her surgery, her pain was at an all-time high. Despite having no bleeding on the continuous Pill, she had missed about 80 days of school since the operation. Her pain was intermittently sharp and stabbing, and radiated from around her pelvis to down her legs. It was aggravated by movement or standing, and as a result she spent most of her days in bed. Her pain was often associated with nausea and she also suffered significant constipation – sometimes needing to strain for up to 20 minutes before she was able to pass a bowel motion. Taking considerable amounts of codeine, which was barely touching the pain, was obviously not helping in this regard.

Her mental health had unsurprisingly taken a dive and she suffered with both anxiety and depression. She felt that endometriosis had taken everything from her and that she was fated to live a life of chronic pain. She also believed that she would have to be on the Pill or have her periods suppressed for her whole life – to 'stop endometriosis from growing back'. Her belief that her endometriosis would probably make her infertile also negatively affected her sense of optimism about the future.

This young woman had been diagnosed with what she was told was a lifelong chronic illness at the age of 13 and the known treatments had already failed. She felt hopeless. Sometimes she thought about suicide but said she would never go through with it because of her strong connection to god and religion. Miranda's mum was despairing, and desperate to have her happy, carefree daughter back.

At Miranda's very first appointment, I was able to explain to her and her mum the science of chronic pain and how when pain persists it has very little to do with an actual stimulus and much more to do with the pain pathways becoming hypersensitive to any sensation in the body. Because her brain was misinterpreting safe signals as dangerous, and in an effort to protect the body from producing more pain signals, Miranda felt more pain when she moved – so she stopped moving. This immobilisation likely led to a tight pelvic floor prone to muscle spasm and constipation (passing a bowel motion through a pelvic floor as hard as concrete is extremely difficult!), and as the cycle continued to feed itself, her body and brain had become more and more conditioned to feel pain.

Her daily pain likely had nothing to do with endometriosis at this point and everything to do with her nervous system and pelvic floor. Identifying, naming and explaining what was going on in her body to produce so much pain was therapeutic in itself. She had answers at last, and could begin to address each factor one by one – like peeling back the layers of an onion to reveal the person she was meant to be when she felt safe in her body.

Miranda left my office that day with four things: a plan to see a pelvic floor physiotherapist to help her work on relaxing her pelvic floor muscles; a neuromodulating medication to turn down the sensitivity in her pain pathways instead of the opiates she had been taking; a referral to a dietician to help with increasing fibre and reducing inflammation through her diet; and a referral to a pain psychologist to work on mindfulness and assist her in retraining her nervous system to return to a sense of safety.

A 360-degree approach like this can feel overwhelming and seem expensive at first glance, but it's often far less expensive and more effective than surgery or a lifetime of medications and missed school or work days. The earlier in a woman's journey she realises that pain is a whole-body, environment and cultural issue, the better the outcome and the less expensive it will be in the long run – both for her and for society.

When Miranda returned to see me three months after her first visit, she was like a different young woman. She lived with her loving, supportive family on their asparagus farm in the country and came bearing a big box of the most beautiful verdant asparagus as a thankyou present. As an obstetrician delivering babies I was used to getting bottles of champagne and boxes of chocolate, but never anything as earthy and beautiful as bunches of home-grown asparagus.

Miranda had been diligent with her homework and found that everything put together had already made a huge difference to her pain levels and quality of life. She had missed only one day of school in the preceding three months.

Another three months later, Miranda was almost pain-free. She had gone back to playing netball and her team had won a premiership. She was attending school every day and had recently had a wonderful holiday overseas with her family.

Eighteen months after her first visit, Miranda came for a review. She was a normal healthy 15-year-old with no issues. She was no longer seeing the physiotherapist, dietician or psychologist regularly, as she now had learnt all the tools for herself. She came off her neuromodulating drug, although she remained on the Pill.

I saw Miranda again at 17 when, after an intense and stressful year in Year 12, she had noticed more pelvic pain. She had the insight to know that stress, anxiety and lack of sleep and movement were all triggers for the mainly neuroplastic component of her pain. Because she had been so well for the past three years she had forgotten to check in and go back to her tools. She had just one appointment with her physiotherapist and started engaging in more mindfulness exercises and ways to deal with the stress of her final year of high school. This little correction helped very quickly, and Miranda was able to get on top of her pain.

I saw Miranda again when she was 19. She had achieved the marks to study pharmacy at university, had moved to the city, and so far everything was going well. She was able to listen to the language of her body with great precision now and automatically make adjustments if she noticed that her stress was on the verge of causing a pain flare – so much so that she was mostly pain-free and living the life you would expect in your first year out of home and at university.

Her issue this time was that she had noticed over the past few years that her hair was very thin and she wondered whether this could be a side effect of long-term Pill usage. It absolutely can be. Since Miranda had been on the Pill so long, she was terrified of how her body would react if left to its own devices. Would her endometriosis grow back? Would she find herself back in crippling pain? While the Pill can be the right choice for some women, this total distrust and fear of natural menstrual cycles, which is very common when girls are put on the Pill at such a young age, breaks my heart.

All that Miranda remembered about her natural periods was pain. We talked about how when I first met her she had already been on the Pill for almost a year and she still had pain – so the Pill didn't help with her persistent pain at all, it just turned off her hormones, cycle and periods. We talked about how her knowledge of her body and the tools she had now were unrivalled compared to the powerless place she was in back at 13 years of age. We talked about how because of her experience with chronic pain, she had developed the super-power of managing her nervous system and listening to her body, and was able to give it what it needed. She was a different person and she knew that she had come too far to hold on to fear. I also reminded her that she was in charge of her body. She had come to her own conclusion that she wanted to come off the Pill and she was in the driver's seat. If she decided her life was better back on it – she could choose to go back. Nothing was set in concrete. There was nothing to fear.

I recommended some other ways to reduce pain with periods and inflammation overall, including supplements such as ginger, omega-3, magnesium, zinc and curcumin, and we talked about paying attention to diet, movement and stress, and making sure she gave herself time to rest during her period.

When I saw her again almost a year later, Miranda said she had been shocked to find that her periods were not painful at all and completely manageable with the tools she had. Miranda had noticed that her hair was thicker even after a few months off the Pill. She now had a boyfriend and was sexually active, so she wanted to talk to me about non-hormonal contraception.

It almost made me cry to hear Miranda talk about how she was enjoying learning about her cycle. She was excited when she noticed fertile mucous, a sign of ovulation, and happy to know that her body was doing exactly what it was supposed to do. She trusted her body at long last.

Miranda's story illustrates so beautifully how when you take a big-picture approach, healing takes place quickly and is sustainable over a long period. With chronic pain, surgery and hormonal drugs are almost never enough because they are not treating the overarching issue within the nervous system.

Rethinking women's pain

Any sensory experience, not just pain, can be driven or turned up by our nervous system. Things like itch, tinnitus (ringing in the ears), fatigue, the sensation of bloating, and feeling the need to empty the bladder can all be neuroplastic symptoms. Many of these same symptoms are often attributed to endometriosis – especially fatigue, body aches and pains, and bloating. If a woman with endometriosis has any of these symptoms it is proof of pain system hypersensitivity and major nervous system upregulation. These symptoms cannot be cured by surgery and are most likely not directly attributable to having endometriosis lesions but to the nervous system roots making pain more likely in the first place.

This phenomenon can become more complicated for women, because all the action going on inside our pelvis as we menstruate each month exposes us to potentially painful stimuli. The amazing processes of ovulation (the release of an egg from the ovary) and menstruation (shedding the uterine lining to signify the end of one cycle and the beginning of the next) would not occur without the inflammatory chemicals produced by our bodies. But inflammatory chemicals can also stimulate the pain receptors in the pelvis during these times in our cycle, which means that most women experience a change in sensation, some discomfort and even pain for the first few days before, and for day one to two of their period. Period and ovulation pain are examples of nociceptive pain. The sensation of pain is produced by the brain in response to the stimuli – so if there are heavier periods or more whole-body inflammation there may be more pain. But the more conditioned women are to fear the pain of menstruation, the more painful it is likely to be.

We know that most women experience some pain with their periods, so are we doomed to a life of pain because we menstruate? Some think that women have drawn the short straw in biology, that our periods can set us up for a lifetime of suffering and that women's pain has been ignored purely because it has been passed off as 'normal'.

I would argue that if the majority of women do experience some pain with periods and many have some discomfort with ovulation, then some period pain is in fact normal. Any severe pain affecting quality of life needs to be investigated and treated, because often pain is a message from the body that needs deciphering, and suffering is not normal or something to accept. But viewing all sensations around periods and ovulation as a danger sign simply ramps up the fear that something dangerous is occurring in the pelvis and this in turn ramps up pain. The rampant fear and panic about the possibility of endometriosis, in my opinion, may be part of the reason why pain is being reported more often by young women.

Language is absolutely critical. It's not about glossing over the 'pain of being a woman'. There is evidence that the language we use to speak about pain literally changes our experience of pain. The sensations aren't the problem. The stories we've been told about the sensations are the problem.

What if girls (and boys) were taught from a young age to revere their bodies and the incredible feats that go on inside them? What if, instead of fear, we waxed lyrical about ovulation being the incredible act of creating a golden egg each month with the possibility of creating life inside us if we desire? What if, instead of talking about 'crazy hormones', we were taught that as an egg grows, it allows our ovarian hormones to be infused into our bodies like magical elixirs, each casting important health-giving spells throughout our bodies to make us strong and beautiful women? What if, instead of learning that periods are a painful, messy curse, we were told that the nest we have built inside us is falling away to make space for a new egg and a new possibility, and that because of all that we have done in our bodies all month long, this period – these days of bleeding – is our chance to rest and recharge for the month ahead? If girls and women knew the truth of just how miraculous their bodies are, I have no doubt that the tsunami of women I see with persistent pain would slow to a gentle wave.

I believe that the negative attention we are paying to pain in women and pain in general is actually making the problem worse. We know that fear drives pain. If we as a society were to acknowledge menstruating people and provide them with the space and support they may need to properly care for their body, would we see less pelvic pain? Normal period pain is a reminder from our body to slow down and, if we listen, not only is the experience of our period better, but also our overall health.

Instead of chasing endometriosis or vilifying periods we need to become intimately aware of our nervous system and learn how to feel safe in our body. We need to bring the treatment of pelvic pain up to the level of modern pain science, which includes the concept of neuroplasticity and pain system hypersensitivity at its core. If we fail to acknowledge this vital piece of the puzzle, we will be practising Dark Ages medicine and failing women with persistent pain.

Chapter summary

- Persistent pain is almost always due to pain system hyper-sensitivity – not ongoing tissue damage or a structural cause. Although, women with periods, particularly endometriosis, may have a mix of neuroplastic and nociceptive pain.
- The longer pain is left untreated the more likely pain system hypersensitivity will occur.
- Pain is more likely to persist in a person with high levels of fear, stress or past and ongoing trauma.
- If you have pain on most days for longer than 3 months you are likely to have pain system hypersensitivity, and surgery or hormonal medications alone is very unlikely to help.
- Your nervous system is plastic and can be rewired to turn pain down just as it was wired to turn pain up.

8

The autonomic nervous system

To understand how trauma can cause pain, we need to examine the actions of the part of our nervous system called the autonomic nervous system. This overarching, evolutionarily older nervous system, which is responsible for whether we feel safe or in danger, changes our downstream biology and physiology, and helps determine if we feel pain in a given situation and how much. The autonomic nervous system is, in effect, the bridge between our mind, our external environment and our body. The intricate workings of the autonomic nervous system help to connect our experiences, our emotions and our biology – dispelling the myth that pain is down to either mind or body and can't be both.

Understanding how the autonomic nervous system works is vital to understanding the huge link between trauma and stress and the increased likelihood of developing and sustaining chronic pain. Not only will it give you the full picture when it comes to understanding how the body can get stuck in pain – which itself is therapeutic because you finally have an answer – but it also means you gain control and mastery over this important system and learn the tools to find your way back to safety and out of pain.

The human nervous system is extremely complex, but it can be broken down into two predominant parts:

1. the central nervous system, comprising our brain and the spinal cord.
2. the peripheral nervous system, comprising all the nerves in the rest of the body that lie outside the brain and spinal cord.

The peripheral nervous system is then further separated into:

1. the somatic nervous system, which is under our control and helps us move our muscles, walk or speak. Somatic nerves also send information – such as sensory signals from our muscles, skin or bones – back to our brain.
2. the autonomic nervous system.

How the autonomic nervous system works

The autonomic nervous system is our ancient operating system that not only functions on autopilot to control crucial bodily processes such as heart rate, digestion and breathing, but also unconsciously detects danger – within our bodies, in the outside environment and within our interpersonal relationships. Some autonomic nerve fibres also send information from our organs back to our brain. Most of the time, the autonomic nervous system functions almost like it sounds – automatically – without any conscious control or direction. It is controlled by the parts of our brain that process emotion and fear – the amygdala and the reticular activating system. These parts of our brain are constantly scanning our environment for safety; if our brain senses danger, it alerts the autonomic nervous system to change our physiology, which helps us survive in the short term.

The autonomic nervous system is essential to life and to our ability to adapt and survive. It can be broken down into two main components:

1. the parasympathetic nervous system controlled by the vagus nerve – also known as the rest and digest nervous system. The freeze or collapse state is also part of the parasympathetic nervous system.
2. sympathetic nervous system, also known as the fight or flight nervous system.

The parasympathetic nervous system is controlled by the two vagal nerves (one on the right and one on the left) that start in our brain stem and wander down the back of the neck into the chest, where they merge together to reach the lungs and heart, and then down to the abdomen and digestive tract, with some fibres even reaching the uterus and cervix. This nerve bundle is called the vagus nerve. 'Vagus' is Latin for 'wanderer' and reflects the way this incredibly important nerve wanders around the body affecting so many of our bodily processes. More than 80 per cent of the messages travelling along the vagus nerve are heading from the body to the brain.

Polyvagal theory

In my view, polyvagal theory, proposed in the mid-1990s by Dr Stephen Porges, an American neuroscientist and psychologist, is the best explanation for the way our nervous system works. In polyvagal theory, there are three components to the autonomic nervous system – two belonging to the vagus nerve and the parasympathetic nervous system, and one to the sympathetic nervous system:

1. ventral (i.e. front) vagal – governing connection, which evolved only in mammals around 200 million years ago (parasympathetic).
2. sympathetic – hyperarousal (fight or flight), which evolved around 400 million years ago.
3. dorsal (i.e. back) vagal – hypoarousal (freeze, collapse, shutdown) – evolved around 500 million years ago (parasympathetic).

Most of the time in a healthy functioning person, the three systems are in balance, which enables a state of health and wellbeing. While the sympathetic nervous system drives our heart to beat (like the accelerator in a car) and controls blood pressure by constricting blood vessels, the parasympathetic nervous system works to slow down the heart. This is known as the 'vagal brake' and keeps things working optimally. The balance between the sympathetic and parasympathetic systems, called the vagal tone, can be measured by heart rate variability. If a person is in good health they tend to have higher heart rate variability, representing high vagal tone, whereas if it is low, it is often a sign of chronic stress and that sympathetic activity is higher than vagal activity. The incredible flexibility and ability of our nervous system to respond to danger means that it can shift into survival mode so that we can literally survive in times of danger and stress.

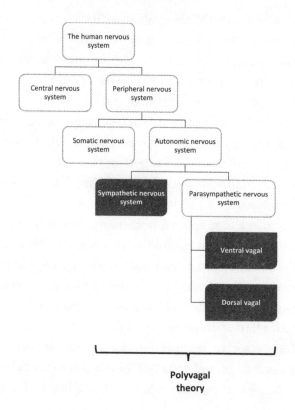

The ventral vagal state

This is our place of safety and connection. It's unique to mammals and the newest nervous state from an evolutionary perspective. When we're in a predominantly ventral vagal state we feel safe, alert, curious, creative, and connected to ourselves, to others and the world around us. From a biological point of view, this state allows for healthy digestion, improved intestinal motility, an optimal gut microbiome, blood supply to skin and extremities, a healthy functioning immune system, lowered inflammation, and the ability for the body to repair and restore itself. When we are here, we feel safe and are not on high alert for danger. This means that sensations from within our body are less likely to be perceived by our brain as dangerous and thus chronic pain is less likely. The ventral vagal can be stimulated by deep breathing, soothing sound, singing or chanting, nature and also safe touch.

The sympathetic nervous system state

The sympathetic nervous system is activated when our nervous system senses danger. It is a protective or survival response. The limbic system in our brain – a primitive part of our brain associated with danger and fear – is activated and in turn stimulates what we call the hypothalamic–pituitary–adrenal axis. This sends signals from the brain to the adrenal glands (small walnut-sized glands that sit on top of each kidney) so that they make our stress hormones – adrenaline and cortisol – which switch us into fight or flight or mobilisation.

Picture a zebra that spots a lion on the horizon and suddenly takes flight, or the rush of adrenaline you might feel if your child or dog suddenly bolted onto a road. Adrenaline makes our heart beat faster, constricts blood vessels to increase blood pressure, shunts blood to our vital organs and muscles, makes our blood stickier to help it clot faster if we're attacked, and makes our muscles tense and contract in preparation for action. It also mobilises sugar from our liver and into our bloodstream to help fuel our fight or flight. When our life is actually in danger, this switch to our sympathetic nervous system state confers an obvious survival advantage by giving us the resources to fight off an attacker or escape a dangerous threat.

In a healthy, regulated system, we can move back into our ventral vagal state when the threat passes, but when we're chronically stressed or have experienced trauma we can get stuck in this survival state. Signs of being stuck in this state of hypervigilance are heightened anxiety, frustration, anger, irritability or restlessness. When we're in this state, we can't seem to relax even if there's no obvious danger. Our connection to self and others is lost. Our concentration and ability to focus mindfully can be impaired. In this state many people see danger everywhere, including – you guessed it – from within the body.

Effects on brain: In this state the brain is much more likely to misinterpret safe signals as dangerous and produce a pain sensation. As we've seen, this pain can cause further fear and stress and then more pain in a vicious feedback loop.

Effects on muscle: Prolonged flight or fight states on a physical level can also lead to more pain through the protective response of contracted muscles – particularly the pelvic floor muscles. When these are in a constant state of contraction, they can become tense and more likely to go into painful spasm – often felt as severe stabbing pelvic pains. A good example of the connection between the sympathetic nervous system and the pelvic floor is what dogs do with their tails when they are scared. From an evolutionary point of view, we all used to have tails and the pelvic floor muscles controlled what the tail would do – stand up straight, wag, or tuck under. Think of a puppy dog when it is scared – it will automatically tuck its tail under as its pelvic floor contracts. Human pelvic floors do exactly the same thing when their sympathetic nervous system activates in fear – but without the tail to show us. Instead we end up with tense and contracted pelvic floor muscles.

Effects on gut: Sympathetic activation can cause impaired digestion and gut microbiome disruption, which can in turn lead to increased leaky gut and immune dysregulation. This not only causes more digestive symptoms – such as bloating, pain, diarrhoea and reflux – but research shows that chronic stress states (likely through this gut–immune system connection) cause more autoimmune disease and could be linked to the role of bacterial LPS and its activation of TLR4 cells which amplify pain and neuroinflammation driving persistent pain (see Chapter 3). Chronic stress also activates immune system receptors that have been implicated in endometriosis and chronic pain states.

In fact, a recent study on rats showed that exposure to stress can even accelerate endometriosis growth through the adrenaline receptors on endometriosis cells. Rats exposed to high levels of stress grew larger endometriosis lesions and displayed greater pain behaviours, while rats that had lower stress and a happy, enriched environment had more regression of endometriosis lesions and showed lower pain behaviours.

Effects on gut and muscles reinforce chronic pain by bottom-up signalling – i.e. giving more information to the brain that there is danger, thereby the brain produces more pain in a bid to protect the body.

The dorsal vagal state

This is also a protective state, activated when we experience either chronic or ongoing stress or an extreme danger. It is our most primitive survival response. Think of how a lizard might freeze when you come across it or how a turtle pulls its head into its shell and immobilises until the threat of danger passes. In humans this can feel like burnout, dissociation, shame, numbness, hopelessness and shutdown. This state can often come about after prolonged flight or fight or when someone has experienced such ongoing or severe trauma that they feel trapped with no way out. Emotionally, it can feel like going through the motions, not being really present, and being unable to connect with self, let alone others. Another manifestation is 'friend or fawn', which can look like 'people pleasing' or placating people at the expense of your own needs.

Whatever the expression, people in the dorsal vagal state can feel disconnected from their bodies.

This state can be a highly successful strategy for surviving an unimaginable trauma, but if someone gets stuck there when the threat has passed, it can inhibit them from being present for their lives, let alone experiencing joy, connection and meaning. Many highly traumatised people seem flat, with blunted facial expressions and voices, and find it difficult to make eye contact. Biologically their bodies are in conservation mode. Their metabolism becomes low to conserve energy, meaning that weight gain is likely, and energy is only spent on the most vital bodily processes. They often report feeling physically exhausted with no energy. Again, this is a protective response, learned in the face of seemingly unrelenting stress. Their immune function is suboptimal, inflammation is high and their body has no energy to spare for recovery and repair.

Because this state is defined by immobilisation, pelvic floor muscles that are not moving will stay tight and dysfunctional, and the avoidance of movement 'in case it hurts' exacerbates pelvic floor tension and reinforces to the brain that any sensations are dangerous, leading to more pain.

Digestion is also impaired in this state, which reduces hunger cues, intestinal motility and even salivation. Irritable bowel symptoms are common in both the sympathetic and dorsal vagal survival states. In fact, it was Elissa Robins, my amazing colleague and dietician – who treats clients with IBS (irritable bowel syndrome) through the lens of the nervous system – who first introduced me to the concept of polyvagal theory. She, along with many other experts, had long realised that IBS was a disorder of the gut–brain axis – specifically the vagus nerve and sympathetic pathways. In fact, the newest science on IBS – which is commonly suffered by women with endometriosis or pelvic pain – recommends treatment with 'gut hypnotherapy' and other therapies for rewiring neural pathways.

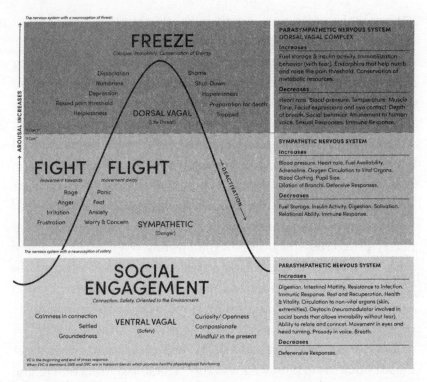

The nervous system with a neuroception of threat:

FREEZE
Collapse, Immobility, Conservation of Energy.

Dissociation
Numbness
Depression
Raised pain threshold
Helplessness

Shame
Shut-Down
Hopelessness
Preparation for death
Trapped

DORSAL VAGAL
(Life Threat)

FIGHT / FLIGHT
movement towards / movement away

Rage
Anger
Irritation
Frustration

Panic
Fear
Anxiety
Worry & Concern

SYMPATHETIC
(Danger)

AROUSAL INCREASES

DEACTIVATION

The nervous system with a neuroception of safety:

SOCIAL ENGAGEMENT
Connection, Safety, Oriented to the Environment.

Calmness in connection
Settled
Groundedness

VENTRAL VAGAL
(Safety)

Curiosity/ Openness
Compassionate
Mindful/ in the present

VC is the beginning and end of stress response.
When VVC is dominant, SNS and DVC are in transient blends which promote healthy physiological functioning.

PARASYMPATHETIC NERVOUS SYSTEM
DORSAL VAGAL COMPLEX

Increases

Fuel storage & insulin activity. Immobilization behavior (with fear). Endorphins that help numb and raise the pain threshold. Conservation of metabolic resources.

Decreases

Heart rate. Blood pressure. Temperature. Muscle Tone. Facial expressions and eye contact. Depth of breath. Social behavior. Attunement to human voice. Sexual Responses. Immune Response.

SYMPATHETIC NERVOUS SYSTEM

Increases

Blood pressure. Heart rate. Fuel Availability. Adrenaline. Oxygen Circulation to Vital Organs. Blood Clotting. Pupil Size. Dilation of Bronchi. Defensive Responses.

Decreases

Fuel Storage. Insulin Activity. Digestion. Salivation. Relational Ability. Immune Response.

PARASYMPATHETIC NERVOUS SYSTEM

Increases

Digestion. Intestinal Motility. Resistance to Infection. Immunic Response. Rest and Recuperation. Health & Vitality. Circulation to non-vital organs (skin, extremities). Oxytocin (neuromodulator involved in social bonds that allows immobility without fear). Ability to relate and connect. Movement in eyes and head turning. Prosody in voice. Breath.

Decreases

Defensive Responses.

Polyvagal chart
Adapted from Ruby Jo Walker (LCSW), Southwest Trauma Training, swtraumatraining.com, 2023

Awareness as the path to healing

While it sounds like we should all aim to hang out in ventral vagal at all times, that's neither possible nor desirable. We need the three pieces of the autonomic nervous system puzzle to make us the incredibly flexible and adaptable creatures we are. They all have a purpose when it comes to helping us survive and experiencing wellbeing.

It's also possible to experience positive sensations in the sympathetic and dorsal vagal states if we can decouple them from fear. There are healthy emotions we can feel in these states – as long as we have the flexibility to return to our ventral vagal state for safety. For example, we need our sympathetic nervous system and mobilisation pathways to help when we're running, exercising intensely or dancing – all of which are wonderful for our health and are a healthy part of completing the stress-response cycle so that you don't get stuck. When dorsal vagal is operating in balance and doesn't flip into shutdown, it's the part of the vagus nerve that controls healthy digestion. The aim is to have an awareness of our nervous system state and to develop the ability to move easily between states – without getting stuck in a prolonged survival state that can make chronic disease more likely.

NEUROCEPTION, INTEROCEPTION AND CHRONIC PAIN

Neuroception is the term used to describe the way our autonomic nervous system is always listening and watching for danger within our bodies and in our environment. This process is unconscious and beyond our control. Think of neuroception as our internal warning system.

People who have experienced trauma or ongoing stress often have a much more sensitive internal warning system because their bodies have been trained to be on high alert for danger. This is a survival advantage in a dangerous environment, but when the danger has long since passed, supersensitive neuroception begins to sense danger everywhere when there is none.

Interoception is the conscious detection of internal signals in your body, many of which are operated by the autonomic nervous system: your heart racing, your stomach growling, your palms getting sweatier. Interoception is the answer to the question 'How do I feel?' or more precisely 'How do I feel in my body (vs my mind)?'

When someone has experienced trauma and is stuck in fight or flight, they are hypervigilant to all their bodily sensations. The volume on their internal warning dial can be turned up so high that safe sensations from inside the body can be misinterpreted as dangerous and may be perceived as painful.

From here you can see how our unconscious autonomic nervous system state can make us more finely tuned for danger and increase fear. This then changes our brain and sets the scene for the development of chronic pain, because at a cellular level our pain system is poised and on high alert to detect any sensation as potentially dangerous and this is perceived in the body as pain.

The good news here is that if our environment can turn up the sensitivity of our internal danger-detection system, throwing us into a survival state that over time causes harm to our health and sense of wellbeing, then changing our environment and becoming aware of this pattern can turn down the sensitivity. This is the whole point of our flexibility and adaptability as humans. If you have a history of trauma or chronic stress and are now thinking: 'Okay, well this might explain things, but what can I do about it? I can't go back and change the past,' the answer is a lot.

When we understand that the body is so powerful and ingenious it can literally, without being asked, change our physiology to help us survive or cope in a dangerous or difficult situation, we can start to see it in a whole new light and even begin to be grateful for its wisdom and skill at keeping us safe when we needed it to step up. We can begin to view our body as the masterpiece it is.

You are not broken and never were. Your body was exquisitely designed to keep you safe. You are here because of its ability to detect and respond to danger. Instead of berating and hating our body for its perceived faults, polyvagal theory helps us to feel gratitude and compassion for everything our body has done for us.

Getting stuck in a survival or protective state happens when we continue to exist in a highly stressful environment or when we haven't had the opportunity to acknowledge or process a past trauma. Just becoming aware of our nervous system states helps us to understand so much about why we feel the way we do, why we behave the way we do and why our body reacts the way it does. From here we can start to recognise the different states and learn how to easily move back to a place of connection and safety when we notice we are becoming stuck in fight, flight or freeze.

If we can listen to our body, we can learn to recognise what state we are in. This is when **neuroception** and **interoception** become **perception** and enters into our conscious awareness. At this point we have the ability to change our nervous system state and rewire it so that we can more easily anchor ourselves in safety and connection. From a place of awareness remarkable change is possible.

Chapter summary

- The autonomic nervous system, which controls our heart rate, breathing and digestion, also acts as an internal warning system.
- In our safe state, our body is at ease and our physical body can function optimally.
- Our nervous system is capable of changing depending on our environment.
- When we feel unsafe we move into a survival state of fight or flight or freeze, which changes our physiology to help us survive in the short term.
- When we get stuck in these survival states, chronic inflammation, gut and microbiome dysfunction, immune dysfunction and chronic pain become more likely.
- We can learn to notice when we are in a survival state and develop tools to bring us back to safety and where chronic pain is less likely.

9

Trauma and pelvic pain

> **CASE STUDY: CASEY**
>
> A few years ago, my amazing husband (also a gynaecologist and an obstetrician) was on call in the emergency department over the Christmas–New Year period, which is traditionally a terrible time to be sick because your normal doctor is often away on holidays. He was called to see a 28-year-old woman called Casey who had arrived with acute pelvic pain. Fortunately for Casey, my husband had heard me talk nonstop about the huge correlation between pelvic pain in women and a history of trauma.
>
> A week or so earlier, Casey's usual gynaecologist had inserted a Mirena IUD to help with her disabling period pain and daily pelvic pain. Another gynaecologist had removed it for her in emergency even though an ultrasound showed it was placed correctly and indicated no other cause for pain. When this did not help Casey's pain, and neither the emergency doctors nor the gynaecologists could get her pain under control, she was admitted as an inpatient.

When my husband saw her, she had been on the ward for a few days. She was still complaining of 9/10 pain, despite being on a ketamine infusion, anti-inflammatories, paracetamol and other neuromodulating medications as well as opiate drugs if she needed them. My husband could have maintained this status quo until Casey's own doctor returned from holidays, but instead made time to take as much of a history as he could in a shared ward with only a curtain for privacy. He rang me shortly after, telling me he had the feeling that underlying trauma could be contributing to Casey's pain.

The following day Casey came to see me at my clinic – still as an inpatient in the hospital, accompanied by her mum. My husband was finding it difficult to get her home without an ongoing treatment plan and a solid answer for what was causing her pain.

Casey told me that although her menstrual bleeding wasn't particularly heavy, her period pain had been increasing over the past few years but had become significantly worse in the past 12 months – interestingly, after she first saw a gynaecologist.

Her GP had done an ultrasound a year earlier to investigate her period pain and found a 4-centimetre uterine fibroid. Uterine fibroids of that size and in the wall of the uterus (not projecting into the uterine cavity) are extremely common, occurring in a third of women, and usually don't cause pain. But the gynaecologist she was referred to advised a laparoscopy to remove the fibroid and to check for endometriosis. The laparoscopy showed no endometriosis and the fibroid was cut out. Casey was then prescribed the oral contraceptive Pill in an effort to stop her periods and hence her pain.

Casey told me that after this surgery her pain became continuous and almost daily. She had ongoing breakthrough bleeding (common with the Pill) and pain that bothered her all the time. She had seen a different gynaecologist who changed the type of Pill she was on for a few months, but her mood worsened, the breakthrough bleeding continued and her pain was still distressing.

A few weeks before her hospital admission for acute pain, Casey underwent a hysteroscopy – a procedure where a tiny camera is inserted into the uterus via the vagina to look for any other cause for abnormal bleeding. She had the Mirena IUD inserted at the same time with the aim of suppressing the growth of the endometrial lining and reducing bleeding. Instead it provoked an intense pain flare that she found impossible to get on top of and that left her feeling completely broken. She felt like she had been thrown in the too-hard basket, on every medication under the sun until someone thought of something to do with her.

As she sat before me with her mum, Casey told me she'd had enough. She was ready for a hysterectomy. She felt she had tried everything that was offered to her as a solution and that removing her uterus and what she felt was at the heart of her pain would be the only thing that could help her now.

I started by listening to her. Instead of asking more about her periods or her uterus or her previous treatments, I asked her about her life. Casey was the only child of supportive, loving parents. She described herself as awkward at school and someone who always had trouble making friends. She was badly bullied during both primary and high school. There were times during high school when she coped with the sadness brought on by the rejection of her peers by engaging in cutting and other self-harm.

She admitted to feeling 'disgusting' and afraid of being vulnerable because of her history of rejection at school. Casey went on to join the army. Her experience in army training became an intensified version of her time at school – with bullying and the pressures of meeting the physical targets taking their toll. She felt lonelier than ever, despite being around people all the time.

When I asked Casey if she had ever experienced any other trauma, she looked down at her feet and fiddled with the hospital ID band on her wrist. I asked if she needed her mum to leave the room and she said, 'It's okay. Mum knows.' During her time in the army she was raped and sexually assaulted on more than one occasion. These events obviously left her completely traumatised, but when she spoke about it to her superiors, it was swept under the carpet and the bullying became even worse, resulting in her leaving the army.

She felt like a failure, like it was her fault, that she couldn't hack it and that she wasn't worth protecting or having an authority figure stand up for. Her mental health took a turn for the worse. Although her workplace was supportive, she felt she was on thin ice after so much time off with her pelvic pain over the past year. This made her feel even more broken. She had few friends outside her family, and she was in an awful place thinking that all that had happened to her, all of the cruelty and abuse she had endured, was her fault. She had no idea why her body was betraying her, and this contributed to her feeling of being totally dysfunctional.

This was the first time a gynaecologist had asked Casey about her mental health, the experiences that had shaped her and whether she had experienced sexual trauma. I asked her if anyone had assessed her pelvic floor muscles and she said they had not. I asked if she felt comfortable enough for me to gently assess her for any pelvic floor muscle tension, explaining that if these muscles were very tight – likely as a result of her previous trauma, both sexual and medical – they could be a big factor in her pelvic pain. She allowed me to do a gentle examination, which revealed obvious pelvic floor muscle tension and tightness.

I told Casey and her mum that I was confident her pain was due to an upregulated nervous system, which in turn had caused her pelvic muscles to become so tight that they could easily go into spasm, causing acute sharp pelvic pain. I told her that she was not broken. Her nervous system had become so dialled up because, after a lifetime of chronic stress and after experiencing sexual trauma where she feared for her life, her body was on constant high alert for danger – both in the environment around her and within her own body.

The volume on her pain signals had been turned up to 10/10, so that previously benign or safe sensations in her body were being misinterpreted by her brain as dangerous – leading to increased pain sensations to any potential stimulus such as a period, an operation, insertion of an IUD, or even a stressful day or less sleep than usual. Casey was unable to pursue joy, pleasure or connection because she was stuck in the fight, flight or freeze part of her nervous system that only cares about survival.

I also explained that because the only way her trauma seemed to be recognised or paid attention to by those in authority was for it to manifest as physical pain, this is where her attention unconsciously went to. When she turned up to the emergency department in pain, she was cared for (the first few times). In contrast, when she spoke up to the authority figures in the army about her rape, she was ignored.

This was the first time in Casey's experience that her actual pain was validated. It didn't take an operation. It didn't take yet another contraceptive drug to turn off her hormones – which was the reason for her ongoing dysfunctional bleeding. It was never her body. It was the band-aid treatment for her pain causing a new symptom. All it took was simply listening to her story.

For the first time, Casey could see the link between what had happened over the course of her life to leave her body feeling so unsafe and the manifestation of her physical symptoms. Her body was far from broken. In fact, it was doing exactly what evolution dictated it do when it felt in danger.

Unfortunately, Casey was stuck in this perpetual state of feeling unsafe, leading to a chronically upregulated nervous system and a host of physical symptoms that were causing her to suffer more.

I could see the sense of relief on Casey's face as we talked through all this. It took a few hours to capture her history and explain to her what I felt was contributing to her pain, but at the end of it, she had some answers. She didn't want a hysterectomy any more (just yet) and she trusted me when I said I thought she could get better with the right help and support and knowledge of her own body.

Instead of going back to the hospital that day, Casey had an initial session with my wonderful pelvic floor physiotherapy colleague to help with pelvic floor muscle relaxation. I gave Casey a plan to stay on only one of her neuromodulating drugs, which would turn the volume down on her pain sensations while she was working though everything. I recommended using some rectal Valium suppositories to help with relaxing her pelvic floor further and prevent painful spasm while she worked with the physiotherapist to do it herself. We also talked about working with her psychologist on unpacking her sexual trauma and the aftermath.

I reminded Casey that some of this work would be hard and that it would take time. She wasn't born with a dialled-up nervous system – it happened because of what she was exposed to. Her entire body was plastic and had adapted to a dangerous environment, but this had become maladaptive over time. Now she knew that if her nervous system could adapt to an unsafe environment, it could adapt to a safe environment. Plasticity is amazing.

I've now been working with Casey for almost two years. Her healing journey has had its ups and downs – real, deep healing always does – but she has moved out of her mum and dad's house and is living by herself. She has had the courage to make a formal complaint to the army about the way her sexual assault was handled, to finally make herself be heard and stand up for herself and for other women who may have been in similar positions.

Casey attends regular support groups for ex-army officers and has grown her own social group around this. She attends the gym and takes pleasure in riding her bike along the river. She has attended our peer support group for women with pelvic pain and trauma, which along with therapy has taught her more about how her nervous system works and how to remodel it through a new lens of safety.

She continues to engage with her support team, which includes her physiotherapist, psychologist, psychiatrist, gynaecologist and peer support group. She asks for help when she needs it, but if she does have a pain flare she can calm her nervous system and wait for it to pass. She no longer has daily debilitating pain. She no longer needs the emergency department because she knows and trusts her own body.

She has a manageable period every month. She is still working on being comfortable with her own body, but the fact that she has got to a point in her journey where she feels safe enough to even go there is huge.

Casey's story is not an isolated one. In fact, almost every woman I see in my practice who has developed chronic pain has a history of trauma and/or chronic, poorly managed stress.

The link between trauma and pain

By suggesting that many of my patients' pain is in large part the result of significant trauma, am I harking back to the days of telling women they are crazy, that there's nothing wrong with them and it's all in their heads? Is there any scientific evidence linking trauma and pain?

Absolutely not and absolutely yes!

As it turns out, the research on trauma and early life experience is really taking off now, and although there's still a long way to go, considerable evidence is mounting up to support my observations in the clinic.

The Adverse Childhood Experiences (ACE) study

The Adverse Childhood Experiences (ACE) study was a large study that took place in the United States during the 1990s. It's worth spending some time on because I believe it was a landmark study, and the first to prove an association between trauma and physical and mental health. One of the principal researchers, Dr Vincent Felitti, was running a weight-loss program for an obesity clinic in the US Department of Preventive Health in the 1980s. One woman who had lost a significant amount of weight in the early part of the program regained the weight a few months later. She explained to him that she had initially put on 105 pounds (48 kilograms) after she was raped at the age of 23. When she started to lose weight in the program, she began noticing the positive attention of men. The fear of violence and her need to feel safe outweighed her desire to be seen as a more socially acceptable size, so she put the weight back on. She said: 'Overweight is to be overlooked, and that's the way I need to be.' At that point, Dr Felitti understood that for many of his patients weight gain was a protective solution to problems that had previously never been discussed with anyone. Some researchers at the Centers for Disease Control (CDC) saw him speak about his findings and as a result the ACE study was born.

The original study involved surveying more than 17,000 people about their experiences of childhood abuse, neglect, family dysfunction, household problems and later-life health and wellbeing. They were asked about eight categories of trauma:

- three categories for personal abuse – including recurrent physical abuse, recurrent emotional abuse or sexual abuse
- four categories related to growing up in a dysfunctional family – including where a family member was an alcoholic or drug

user; where a family member was in prison; where someone in the family was chronically depressed, mentally ill or suicidal; or where there was violence towards the mother

- one category about parental separation, divorce or where a parent was lost to the child in some way when they were growing up.

If participants answered no to all experiences they had an ACE score of zero, if yes to one experience, an ACE score of one, and so on. The higher the score, the more traumatic events you had experienced.

The original study followed up the participants for at least five years, to compare their childhood experiences with ongoing adult pharmacy costs, visits to the doctor and emergency department, hospitalisations and death.

The researchers found that adverse childhood events were very common. Around half of the study population had experienced at least one ACE. One in four had experienced two or more and one in eight had experienced at least four. Girls were typically more likely to experience sexual abuse, while boys were more likely to experience physical abuse. It's worth noting that this study was more than 74 per cent white, and later breakdowns of the data showed that typically non-white, lower socioeconomic participants and women were more likely to report multiple ACEs.

The big significance of the study was that it found that the higher the ACE score the more likely you were to suffer from chronic disease, both physical and mental, as an adult, including addiction and suicide. It might sound obvious that being poorly treated as a child would lead to things like depression, anxiety, PTSD and substance abuse, but what was not as clear up to this point was that exposure to developmental trauma also had a strong association with chronic physical illness, such as heart disease, respiratory disease, type 2 diabetes and cancer.

Later studies have shown that early life trauma and stress are also associated with conditions such as polycystic ovarian syndrome (PCOS), premenstrual dysphoric disorder (an extreme form of premenstrual syndrome), autoimmune disease and even an increased susceptibility to infection.

Chances of disease development after childhood trauma

Condition	Increased likelihood after four adverse experiences
Heart disease	2.9 times
Cancer	1.6 times
Chronic obstructive pulmonary disease (COPD; lung disease)	Almost 4 times
Depression	4.6 times
Suicide	12.2 times
Smoking	2 times
Alcoholism	7 times
Heroin/crack use	9.7 times

The original ACE study made it clear for the first time that what happens to us – especially in early life – matters. Our experiences shape us, not just emotionally and in the way we relate to self and others; they literally make physical disease in adult life more likely. The original ACE study also showed an increased association between higher ACE scores and the pain conditions fibromyalgia, lower back pain, migraine, facial and jaw pain, pregnancy-related pain and, you guessed it, pelvic pain and pain with sex.

The types of exposures more likely to predispose people to pain conditions were:

- abuse – physical, emotional and sexual
- neglect – emotional and physical
- household dysfunction.

Studies into trauma and chronic pelvic pain

A multitude of studies has found an increased likelihood of chronic pelvic pain in women who have experienced trauma in childhood. A 2018 study even found that women who had experienced physical and sexual trauma in childhood were more likely to have been diagnosed with endometriosis. This is interesting, but what I would like to see is whether abuse history is correlated with an even higher number of laparoscopies for *pelvic pain* even with no endometriosis diagnosed. As we know, pelvic pain is more relevant than superficial endometriosis.

This is borne out by a 1998 study that showed chronic pelvic pain was more prevalent in women who had suffered sexual or physical trauma and neglect. These women also had measurable differences in their levels of stress hormones, suggesting that early life trauma and a subsequent chronically stressed state can alter the body's stress-response system.

A large study published in 2020 looking at more than 48,000 children and adolescents, found that ACEs are strongly associated with the development of chronic pain, and the greater the number of ACEs the stronger the association. More than 18 per cent of children with more than four ACEs had chronic pain. It's interesting to note that this study did not ask about physical or sexual trauma, but was more focused on financial hardship, bullying, discrimination and family dysfunction. If we accounted for all the children who have experienced the big-T traumas of physical or sexual abuse, the numbers would no doubt be higher.

A 2022 systematic review concluded that there was a significant association between the number of ACEs and period pain, and that sexual abuse and resultant PTSD were the ACEs most strongly associated with pelvic pain, period pain and pain with sex. The same group published a paper in 2023 showing a link between self-reported endometriosis symptoms such as pain and a history of trauma. Interestingly, they found this link between papers looking at pain irrespective of whether endometriosis was found at laparoscopy but not that laparoscopically confirmed endometriosis was always associated with trauma. Another piece of evidence that may suggest endometriosis, on its own, isn't the problem but the upregulated nervous system caused by stress and/ or trauma that leads to pain.

This theory was borne out in a 2023 study showing that severe pelvic pain is associated with sexual abuse experienced during childhood or adolescence, irrespective of the presence of endometriosis. This study concluded that taking a complete history, including the experience of sexual trauma, in people presenting with pelvic pain was important to provide comprehensive care to patients.

It certainly feels like the tide is turning, and I am hopeful that what happens to girls and women and the long term effects it has on their lives is starting to receive the attention it deserves, rather than continuing to be ignored or swept under the carpet.

Gender differences in pain and trauma

Studies have looked at gender differences in both the number and types of ACEs girls and boys are exposed to and later effects on adult health. Generally, most studies have found that girls usually experience a higher number of ACEs with one study showing that 29 per cent of girls experienced 6+ ACEs compared with 14 per cent of boys. Girls are typically more likely to experience sexual abuse, while boys are more likely to experience physical abuse. In terms of the effects on their health in later life, most studies show that girls are likely to internalise their experiences with a greater prevalence of anxiety, depression, complex PTSD, and somatic complaints such as pain and obesity. Whereas boys are more likely to externalise their trauma – with greater risk of problems at school, criminality and violence.

The obvious theories are all about what changes at puberty between the sexes. Girls start menstruating, their oestrogen levels increase and then fluctuate, boys' levels of testosterone leave women's in the dust. All of these biological things do indeed happen and may play a part in the higher incidence of pelvic pain in women. After all, we do have a potentially painful stimulus in periods each month. But is it really as simple as periods and hormonal differences? In this model of biological reductionism – where women are born with the inferior and problematic version of the human body – is it reasonable that all women should develop persistent pain just by virtue of our second-rate biology?

My interpretation is that women have more pain because they are more likely to be mistreated and, in particular, sexually abused as children and throughout their lives. They are expected to pretend they don't have a female body if they want to excel in a capitalist society – there is no time or room for a body that needs to rest in such a society. It might not be explicitly said, but the fact that our culture creates no room, let alone nurtures or celebrates a bleeding and cycling person, demonstrates to young women that their bodies are less-than and what makes them different should be ignored, turned off or feared. They, alongside their brothers, are living in a toxic environment contributed to by their poor diet, lack of sleep, copious screen time, lack of nature and lack of joyful movement and play. Girls and women are more likely to internalise their trauma and develop a chronically stressed nervous system as a result of developmental trauma and ongoing chronic stress, which make potentially mildly painful stimuli like the inflammation from a period much more painful.

I have already spoken extensively about how, despite what we like to believe about the status of women in the West, women are living under an intensely patriarchal society that demands that women pretend they don't have ovaries to 'succeed' on the linear gauge on which we measure success. Women are conditioned to push down their pain – and I don't just mean physical pain, but the pain of not being allowed to fit in to a patriarchal world and the pain of suppressing their stories of abuse, objectification and the impossible task of pretending that they don't have hormonal ebbs and flows and physiological changes across the month.

As the physician and author Gabor Maté says so eloquently in his book *The Myth of Normal*: 'Women are targeted by a culture that does not honour, but demeans, distorts and even impels people to suppress who they are.' He says that, 'Early childhood mechanisms of self-suppression are reinforced by persistent, gendered social conditioning. Many women end up self-silencing, defined as the tendency to silence one's thoughts and feelings to maintain safe relationships.'

The chronic suppression of one's authentic self reinforces a lack of safety – in that it is not safe to be fully expressed. In this way many women are living in a chronic survival or danger state – where chronic illness including pain is more likely. Not only do women who have experienced more trauma experience more pain, there is evidence that their very immune systems are altered to constantly be on high alert.

Bessel van der Kolk, renowned psychiatrist, trauma specialist and author of *The Body Keeps the Score*, has talked about how he noticed a large proportion of the women he was working with who had experienced sexual assault had developed auto-immune conditions. He was able to study the immune cells of these patients with the help of an immunologist colleague at his university and found that women who had suffered sexual abuse had overactive CD45 cells compared to controls. I find this fascinating and amazing, but not surprising because of my knowledge of how trauma affects our nervous system and hence all the other systems of the body. It means that not only did these women feel unsafe and were living in a constant state of danger, but their immune cells were on edge and dialled up to overactivity to respond to any sign of danger. Unfortunately, if our immune system is chronically heightened in the absence of disease, it begins to turn inwards and respond to our own cells as if they were dangerous. This is auto-immune disease and it is well-known to be increased in women in general, and women with trauma more so.

How does trauma lead to pain?

Thirty years of research clearly demonstrate that early life trauma is associated with poor health outcomes in later life – including a higher risk of developing chronic pain. But how? Changes in cortisol or stress hormone production and their effect on the brain are part of the story, but like everything when it comes to pain, it's more complex than that. A recent study looking at the impacts of early life stress in rats, as well as the impact of a high-fat, high-sugar diet, revealed fascinating insights into the potential ways trauma leaves long-lasting effects on the body.

The researchers divided the rats into four groups – a control group fed a normal diet and allowed to have normal care from their mothers, and three study groups – one fed a high-fat, high-sugar diet; one exposed to maternal separation (mimicking early life trauma); one fed the poor diet and also separated from their mothers. They looked at levels of anxiety, response to pain by exposure to hot and cold stimuli, and recovery after an operation to a paw. They also took functional MRI brain images.

Rats from all three non-control groups exhibited increased anxiety behaviour, and altered pain responses both before and after surgery. Brain MRIs showed that both poor diet and maternal separation affected the maturity of the brain, with changes in brain volume and in the parts of the brain related to fear and pain processing. The effects of maternal separation and poor diet were cumulative, resulting in exacerbated pain sensitivity and increased brain and nervous system changes. This work is important, because, unlike the human studies, it shows definitive cause and effect rather than just suggests an association.

These findings are huge, but they were built on decades of research exploring the link between early stress and poor health in later life. Previous work on adolescent pain conditions showed that exposure to ACEs such as neglect, abuse and household dysfunction increased inflammation in the brain. Other human studies have also demonstrated that exposure to ACEs is associated with changes in brain structure and function, especially in parts of the brain associated with physical and emotional pain processing. Mirroring the rat study, a plethora of evidence shows that diets high in processed foods increase inflammation in the body, including the brain, where it leads to structural and functional changes. MRI studies show that poor diets are linked to decreased brain volume compared with good diets. This is no revelation, given we know that diets high in processed food increase the likelihood of heart disease and type 2 diabetes, which both translate into increased risk of dementia later in life.

We know that both stress and a processed diet increase inflammation – by altering our gut microbiome and intestinal mucous layer, resulting in damage to our gut wall and leading to increased intestinal permeability or leaky gut. We looked earlier at the theory that endometriosis occurs when leaky gut leads to bacterial LPS interacting with toll-like receptors (TLR4) and increasing inflammation throughout the body. There is lots of research now that the resultant inflammation can upregulate glial cell activity in the brain which may also be part of the pain amplification process that contributes to the maintenance of persistent pain conditions.

The reality is that not only do children from lower socioeconomic backgrounds have higher rates of childhood trauma, but they also tend to have poorer diets due to limited access to fresh or organic produce and financial strain in their homes. Additionally, as we saw earlier, childhood trauma and the resultant persistent stress are associated with an increased risk of obesity. This may be due to an unconscious need to feel safer by being in a bigger body, but it may also simply be the result of trying to soothe a nervous system stuck in constant flight or fight. We're all familiar with stress or comfort eating. It might be okay every once in a while, but if your nervous system is stuck in a constant state of stress, and eating processed food is your learned way of coping, obesity seems almost inevitable.

There is scientific evidence that stress eating is real. When we initially experience a stressor, our adrenal glands release adrenaline that takes away our appetite, but as stress continues, the release of cortisol causes us to crave sugary and high-fat foods. When we satisfy our cravings, feedback to the brain lowers cortisol levels and leaves us feeling soothed or numbed out. This promotes a pro-inflammatory state in the body, which lies at the root of chronic pain and almost all chronic disease. The combination of stress and poor diet causes these disastrous effects to snowball in later life.

Lives of chronic stress

As dynamic, sophisticated and clever creatures, we have nervous systems with an incredible capacity to adapt and survive in a high-stress environment, and we learn coping strategies to help us feel okay or momentarily safe. Often these coping strategies, which can be effective in the short term, become unhelpful and harmful in the long term. To make matters worse, conventional medicine usually blames people for the way their 'bad choices' cause their own health problems. Simply telling someone to eat more healthily, to exercise more, to feel and express their feelings, or to reduce stress can never be effective if these behaviours were carved into our being as a survival strategy. That's why many patients and their doctors give up. Behavioural change is too hard. Band-aid treatments are given to address symptoms, but they never touch the underlying problem and often lead to troublesome side effects while also perpetuating the underlying state that continues to drive chronic disease.

The current medical paradigm is merely a cog in the wheel of a system that amounts to a biological–environmental mismatch that is making and keeping people in industrialised capitalist societies sick. Setting aside some of the appalling and tragically common violence and abuse that many children are forced to endure, there is also the frequent 'benign neglect' that even children with well-meaning and loving parents often experience.

Families

Our society values work, money, productivity and ever-bigger profit margins more than mothers and childhood and the work of creating a loving, supportive environment for families to grow in safety. Women are told they can have it all, but to do so they need to work like they don't have children and have children like they don't work. They can feel like choosing motherhood and family over career, even for a little while, is somehow failing feminism.

Does this sound familiar to you? You and your partner work and your small children go to childcare. When you come home, you try to fit a day of taking care of the house and kids into an hour before everyone falls on the couch watching Netflix – or more realistically each goes to their separate bedroom and separate screen. You're stressed at work and stressed at home. Healthy eating falls by the wayside because convenience foods are easier and cheap. It's hard to find time for the simple daily rituals of caring for your bodies. Trying to get the kids to all their activities means you have no time for exercise and play yourselves. Fuses become short, along with attention spans and tempers. You feel like you're trying to pour from an empty vessel and have nothing more to give.

Children sense the tension and stress. They feel the lack of attention – even if every minute of their day is scheduled with activities. They watch and they learn what it means to be grown up. Rest and play are for lazy people. There is no space for their nervous systems to rest – to just be. Modern life drives all of our nervous systems into fight, flight or freeze.

Adolescents

I see so many teenage girls who tell me how stressed out they are. Their days at school often start at 6 am. They begin with sports training or music and then, when they finish school, they are on to their next activity. Many girls have afternoons filled with extracurricular activities.

They may do sport several times a day. They're not taught that their hormones change throughout their cycles, causing changes to their metabolism that can alter their exercise endurance, inflammation levels and risk of injury. My stepdaughter told me that her PE teacher said to the class, 'It's okay if you lose your period because of sport.' I was furious! Their bodies are treated like machines. They do not learn that their bodies will be in optimum health if they know the rhythms of their cycle and can find a way to move, rest and eat according to their inner flow state. It's no wonder they burn out. Many of them are on the Pill so that their periods don't get in the way, with possible side effects such as anxiety and depression.

Women who start the Pill in adolescence show the same blunting of the cortisol response as chronically stressed people. In addition, while there is evidence that fluctuating oestrogen levels can lead to more pain, there is also some that shows that the lower oestrogen levels on the Pill can contribute to painful vulval conditions and may be detrimental for pain tolerance. There is even emerging evidence that low-testosterone states (like the one induced on the Pill) may be associated with a greater risk of pain persistence.

After their busy days at school, these girls may arrive home just before dinner and if they're lucky have dinner with family before going off to their bedrooms to study. When they finish at 9.30 or 10 they might 'wind down' with Netflix or talking to friends on social media. The pressure of performing well academically as well as in the sporting arena, and to look like a filtered airbrushed Instagram model is insane. They are rarely getting anywhere near enough sleep and often either eating ultra-processed convenience foods on the run (because there's no time to eat) or engaging in restricted and disordered eating patterns (because there's no time to eat and they need to be a certain size to be loved and accepted).

Often when I send these girls to my physiotherapist, Brooke Dobó, to help them with pelvic floor relaxation, she tells me they can't even breathe properly and have totally dysfunctional movement patterns because their experience with exercise is all about high intensity and 'toning'. Girls think their stomachs should be flat at all times and spend most of their time holding them in and breathing shallowly into the top of their lungs. If humanity is getting to the point that it doesn't even know how to breathe in a way that calms the nervous system, we're in big trouble.

The rates of anxiety and depression among teenage girls have been steadily rising over the past 20 years. A recent report showed that more than 38 per cent of teenage girls have a significant anxiety disorder. This is more than one in three of our girls and they're just the ones seeking help. I've seen many girls who are seeing a psychologist or a psychiatrist to help with their anxiety symptoms. While they often have undergone some form of talk or cognitive behavioural therapy to help with their symptoms, many do end up on antidepressants to manage their symptoms. I'm not anti-medication at all, but very few girls have been told how their autonomic nervous system works and how it can be implicated in anxiety symptoms. They don't know how to work with their nervous system to calm not just their anxiety but also the trickle-down effects of chronic stress, including chronic pain. Anxiety, like pain – and they often go together – is part of the language of our bodies. It's trying to tell you that you can't keep going on like this. Humans are not meant to live like this.

It's time to slow down and listen to our bodies

Even if you don't think you've experienced any trauma, growing up in our stressful society is a trauma too. We're not machines. We're animals whose needs are not being met. To survive we try to adapt by dialling up our sympathetic nervous system in order to keep up with the never-ending pace of life. By the time we reach adulthood, we don't know how to listen to our body. We don't even know how to sit still or in silence. We don't know how to access that part of our nervous system that slows us down, that allows our body to repair, to digest and to recover.

It's no wonder our body forces us to slow down instead. When we have pain or fatigue that doesn't go away, we're made to stop. If teenage girls don't learn how to dial in and dial down now, what will they be like when they have a full-time job, kids, a partner, financial responsibilities, other people to look after? What will their health, and their kids' health look like in 20 years?

Because mainstream medicine fails to recognise the effect our experiences have on our body, conventional treatments are often bound to fail, keep us stuck and make us feel broken. But humans are not broken. They are not lazy. They are not stupid. They are not bad.

We are the product of an environment that's deeply mismatched to our biology. If you have chronic pain and a dialled-up nervous system and a history of trauma, you are amazing. You have survived, thanks to the sophistication of your body and brain. Understanding this is the key to finding your way to the true path of healing.

If people understood how the trauma of being a woman affects the way we cope with periods, we might spend more time celebrating the magnificence of the female body, creating space in society for girls and women to rest during menstruation, and educating them about how stress affects their cycles and their bodies.

As one doctor has written on the effects of childhood trauma: 'Human brains work better when they are allowed to develop in safe and nurturing environments, and human bodies experience less pain when they are allowed to receive input from a healthy brain. When we insist on approaching chronic pain as a purely biomedical phenomenon . . . we consign the patient to suboptimal treatment. That's not acceptable. [They] were mistreated once as children; there is no excuse for history to repeat itself when they become patients.'

There is an unconscious notion that the only way to legitimately rest when we have a period is to have a dreadful disease like endometriosis. If you don't have endometriosis, there is no validation for your unique needs as a woman and you have to soldier on. Is it any wonder our nervous system is screaming at us?

I don't have all the answers. But I do know the answer to most chronic pelvic pain lies in our nervous system, which affects everything else. And I also know that the power to rewire our nervous system is in our hands.

The time is now

Now is the time for doctors to really listen to women's pain and not to turn away when operations fail to solve the problem. I recently saw a woman with chronic pelvic pain who'd had a diagnostic laparoscopy that found no endometriosis. When she asked the surgeon at her post-op review what they thought was causing her pain, they said, 'Your guess is as good as mine.'

CASE STUDY: ROSIE

Rosie, who recently came to my practice, had seen another gynaecologist for pain during and after sex and using tampons. The gynaecologist's letter describing his approach and treatment shocked even me. He completely removed the inner part of the vulva and performed a procedure to widen the vaginal opening so that sex was less painful. He wrote that Rosie was now 'able to manage sex with a reasonable degree of comfort'. Apart from the fact that this was untrue – Rosie continued to have pain with sex, even more so – his casual use of the word 'manage', with no mention of her pleasure, says so much about how women are often viewed when it comes to sex and pain. As far as he was concerned, the problem was fixed. If a man had a painful penis would his doctor ever suggest excision of part of his penis? Of course not – there would be outrage, cries of medical malpractice and abuse.

Unsurprisingly, Rosie had a long history of sexual trauma, complex trauma arising from her relationship with her parents, and ongoing issues with her husband – all of which probably contributed massively to her pain symptoms in the first instance. Her doctor had never asked her about her experiences or helped her join the dots.

Rosie arrived at our clinic to see our physiotherapist, Brooke, and start the work to heal her childhood trauma, understand how pain develops and learn the tools for creating a sense of safety in her body and rewiring her pain pathways. She wrote to Brooke: 'I feel very grateful to have met you and found your clinic. You are the first person I've met that understands everything that I'm saying and thank you for helping me to make sense of it all.'

Trauma-informed care, psychoeducation, physiotherapy, modern pain science and a heart-centred approach should be the standard of care for all women – not something so rare that women are grateful to find it after years of suffering.

Now is the time to address pelvic pain in a way that acknowledges its complexity, that is seeded in cutting-edge science, and that actually gets to the root of the problem.

We must be brave enough to face the truth, we must be strong enough to really hold women's pain and make space for women to exist authentically in the world. We must be ready to tear down the current medical paradigm and create an entirely new approach. I'm ready. Are you coming with me?

Chapter summary

- There is a well-established link between early life trauma and physical and emotional illness including pain in later life.
- Trauma changes our brain, pushes us into survival nervous system states like fight, flight and freeze, which leads to a perpetual perception of danger in the body.
- Being stuck in a survival state increases inflammation, leaky gut, activation of the toll-like receptor which can lead to the neuroinflammation of chronic pain.
- Nervous system dysregulation also leads to alterations in muscular behaviour, breathing patterns, metabolism and puts us on high alert for danger outside and inside the body pain system hypersensitivity.
- The higher rates of traumatic events and the 'go, go, go' of modern life for women contributes to nervous system dysregulation, further driving pain.

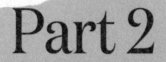

Part 2

A practical pathway
to true healing

10

Reducing inflammation and supporting the immune system

Period pain is an inflammatory event and not to be feared, especially if we can make room for it in our lives.

But a dysregulated nervous system due to unresolved trauma and/or chronic stress can alter the gut microbiome and lead to immune dysfunction that can increase inflammation and lead to more pain. This in turn can create pelvic muscle tightness and dysfunction, which also increases pain. The fear of endometriosis, combined with a nervous system stuck in fight, flight or freeze, primes pain pathways and the brain to keep pain persistent. Over time, this turns up the volume on our pain pathways so that we feel sensitive to every sensation in the body. This can show up as increased pain even on days you don't have a period, extreme pain with periods, and a tendency to headaches, body aches, feeling bloated and fatigue.

The hypervigilance of the fight or flight state means every sensation is amplified, and this is the experience of women with chronic pain. The freeze state can lead to feelings of chronic exhaustion. In both states, digestion is massively impaired, which is why endometriosis is commonly associated with IBS. It's not, as many women believe, the endometriosis lesions that cause the gut issues, it's the overarching nervous system dysregulation leading to more period pain, bloating, gut issues, immune system dysfunction and increased inflammation.

In contrast, when we feel safe in our environment, we're more likely to be in our rest and digest state, where our body is in optimal health, and fear and pain are less likely. This is where we thrive.

I always start by educating women about their bodies and demystifying what's going on each month – not just with their period but throughout their whole cycle – and by teaching them that their periods are not a disconnected part of them. The menstrual cycle is inseparable from the health of the whole woman. Just as our body and mind cannot be separated, neither can the systems within our body or even our relationship with our environment.

Rewriting the narrative of women's bodies and periods creates a sense of safety from the start. I hope that in the future young women start to feel nurtured and revered when they begin their periods, rather than embarrassed, ashamed, inconvenienced and not safe enough to have a period.

If you're the parent or caregiver of a young woman, you can begin to lay the groundwork for this before your daughter gets her period, reframing it not as a curse or something to push through but as a sacred time to rest and be cared for. It's really important to reaffirm that periods can be uncomfortable or even mildly painful for the first few days and that this is normal and not something to be afraid of. Starting from a place of health rather than viewing periods – and the possibility of endometriosis – as a disease state, is a vital first step in setting up young women to stay in their ventral vagal or safe nervous system state, which is far less likely to promote pain. Being there and open to listen to her pain – both emotional and physical – is also incredibly important.

Flipping the script to one of such positivity may not be easy at first. If you see your body as the enemy and have suffered immensely, you may want to throw this book at the wall right now. I don't blame you.

If you're in the early stages of exploring your pain, a comprehensive approach to pain early on can help nip it in the bud and prevent the development of chronic pain. So many young girls see their GP only to be given the options of the Pill or anti-inflammatories. I want to give you *all* the solutions. I barely ever prescribe the Pill for period pain – although I give it as an option – because women and girls do so well after education and other strategies that get to the root causes of period pain: inflammation, immune system dysfunction, gut health, nervous system dysregulation and pelvic floor upregulation.

Simple remedies for initial period pain

A period *is* an inflammatory process and most women experience some discomfort or pain for a few days before and during the first days of bleeding. Excess inflammation can cause more pain, as can our nervous system state, our pelvic floor and our gut health. An abnormally painful period is a sign from our body that we need to look at everything else that can be increasing inflammation or dialling up our nervous system state.

Medications and self-care during a period

It's important to address period pain early to avoid upregulation of pain pathways. If education, self-care and simple measures such as diet, heat and gentle movement are not effective, I would start with some anti-inflammatory herbs and supplements followed by over-the-counter medications. Overuse of non-steroidal medication like Nurofen and Ponstan can worsen gut symptoms and contribute to IBS and leaky gut, so I would usually recommend the following first:

- ginger root capsules (500 milligrams three times a day). Numerous studies have shown these to be as effective as ibuprofen and Ponstan for period pain. Ginger tea is another option.
- heat packs, warm baths, gentle yoga and walking.

- allowing yourself space to take things more slowly and promote the period as a time for real self-care. (See Chapter 18 for a detailed guide.)

If periods are still painful, you could move on to:

- ibuprofen and paracetamol taken regularly. These medications are anti-prostaglandins and help to mop up inflammatory prostaglandins before they can cause pain.
- if periods are heavy, tranexamic acid (Cyklokapron) plus ibuprofen. This combination has been found to be as effective at reducing pain and bleeding as the Pill.

Working on root causes that increase inflammation and fear and dial up pain pathways will also help to reduce the need for regular anti-inflammatory medications in many women. It is important to stop the wind up of pain initially while you get on top of things, as continuous bouts of acute pain are more likely to lead to chronic pain in the future.

Being aware of your lifestyle throughout the month helps set you up for an easy period and reinforces the idea that the way we experience our periods is a reflection of our underlying general health.

A Mediterranean anti-inflammatory diet

A general recipe for a healthy and easeful period is the same as that for a healthy body. While there is no conclusive evidence that one way of eating is better for women with painful periods than another, the quality of our diet does impact our gut microbiome and gut lining. There is no one-size-fits-all endometriosis diet but a wholefood Mediterranean diet has the best evidence for reducing inflammation and, unsurprisingly, it has the best evidence for good health, including a healthy gut microbiota. As endometriosis, pain and IBS have all been linked to an altered gut microbiome – diet is important. Gut health involves many things, one of which is ensuring the healthy mucous lining of the small intestine is working well and the other is that of a healthy gut microbiome.

We know that when the mucous barrier is broken down, the gut can become leaky, allowing unwanted bacteria and other products into the body. Remember that LPS – which has been associated with pelvic pain and endometriosis, can turn on pain by activating TLR4 as we learned in Chapter 3.

Your best bet is to focus on an anti-inflammatory diet high in fibre and prebiotics (which feed the microbiome), polyphenols and good fats such as those in olive oil, and low in trans fats, refined sugar and large amounts of processed, factory-farmed or grain-fed red meat. This advice is applicable to everyone on the planet. In general, our poor, overly processed Western diet laden with simple carbohydrates, sugar and inflammatory fats has played a huge part in the skyrocketing rates of chronic disease. Because our periods and menstrual cycle cannot be separated from the rest of our body, high overall bodily inflammation can show up as more painful periods.

Think about the quality of your period as a report card on the health of the rest of your body, as Dr Lara Briden espouses in her book *Period Repair Manual*. Or like a warning light flashing on your car dashboard, telling you that you need to check under the hood. You're grateful for the warning light because it lets you address the problem promptly rather than getting halfway down the highway and grinding to a halt with smoke billowing from the bonnet.

Severe pain is always a signal that either there is tissue damage or that the brain mistakenly thinks there is danger – and both deserve attention. If we learn to listen with curiosity and without fear, we can deal with issues by addressing their upstream causes. In many cases this not only improves our experience with our periods but can also prevent other health issues in the future. This is another of the many reasons that just using the Pill as a band-aid to treat period problems misses the mark so much of the time.

You may find that following some of the guidelines below will help you maintain good overall health and reduce the burden of inflammation in your body. As a rule, according to Vera dietician Desi Carlos, increasing fibre, and reducing saturated fats and sugar are the cornerstones to improved gut health, a healthy microbiome and decreased inflammation, but an individualised approach with you at the centre of what feels right in your body is THE most important thing.

What to eat

From current research, foods that may help gut health include:
- omega-3 fats, which are anti-inflammatory fats found in olive oil, fish, nuts and seeds
- probiotic foods, such as Greek yoghurt and kefir
- foods high in resistant starches, like cooked and cooled potatoes, oats and rice
- high-fibre foods rich in prebiotics (which feed the microbiome), such as:
  o fruits – particularly berries, which are high in anti-inflammatory polyphenols
  o vegetables – particularly garlic, leeks, onions, asparagus and artichokes
  o legumes – especially lentils
  o grains – especially barley and oats for beta-glucans.

An adequate fibre intake helps support a diverse microbiome. This encourages optimal metabolism and excretion of excess oestrogen, which can be inflammatory and worsen pain symptoms. Having a regular bowel movement can also help decrease bloating, pain and IBS-like symptoms. Aim for a diet that includes at least 30 grams of fibre each day.

An example of a Mediterranean anti-inflammatory diet over the course of a week

- **Red meat** – a 120g serve of grass-fed beef 0–1 times per week (this absolutely makes a difference in reducing pain)
- **Chicken** – two 150g serves of chicken 2 times per week; 4–6 eggs per week
- **Fish** – 150g serve 4–6 times per week – salmon, mackerel, blue eye trevalla, sardines (tinned or fresh)
- **Nuts** – 50g per day: especially walnuts – which are rich in omega 3s, or almonds

- **Dairy** – 30g cheese, 125g yoghurt, 250ml milk, calcium-fortified milk
- **Extra virgin olive oil** – 2–4 tbs per day (include 4–8 olives per day)
- **Fruits** – 2 per day (include a serve of tomato every day)
- **Vegetables** – 3 cups per day
- **Legumes** – 3 cups per week
- **Breads and cereals** – 2–6 serves per day: carbohydrates with lower glycaemic load such as sourdough and unrefined grains
- **Herbs, spices, garlic, onion** – even though some people will report some **gut irritability from garlic and onion**, Desi has never, in practice, seen anyone react to both.

WHAT DOES 30 GRAMS OF FIBRE LOOK LIKE?

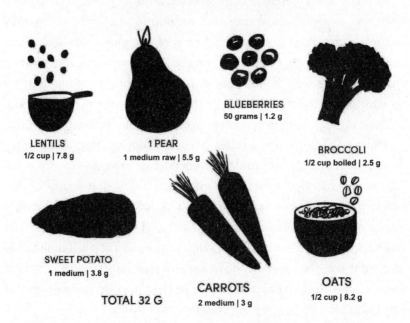

LENTILS
1/2 cup | 7.8 g

1 PEAR
1 medium raw | 5.5 g

BLUEBERRIES
50 grams | 1.2 g

BROCCOLI
1/2 cup boiled | 2.5 g

SWEET POTATO
1 medium | 3.8 g

TOTAL 32 G

CARROTS
2 medium | 3 g

OATS
1/2 cup | 8.2 g

In terms of FODMAP, Desi recommends using it as a diagnostic diet, NOT a permanent diet. She uses it only if symptoms persist after all other processes are exhausted. She believes that following a Mediterranean diet improves symptoms in 9 out of 10 of her clients without resorting to a low-FODMAP diet.

If, with a practitioner, you do decide to remove FODMAP foods, it should be done for 4 weeks maximum. Once symptoms are relieved, changes must be undertaken and then identification of culprit categories conducted. Retesting should be undertaken again after 6 months.

It is IMPERATIVE that a low-FODMAP diet is not followed for extensive periods of time as it may lead to a more dysbiotic effect on gut microbiota and more inflammation.

It should always be undertaken with the guidance of a FODMAP-trained dietician.

A note about dairy and gluten

Desi doesn't recommend a blanket ban on gluten and dairy.

Gluten: Desi recommends coeliac and thyroid testing and if either of these show positive autoantibodies, then she may recommend a trial of a gluten-free diet, as gluten and/or wheat can be inflammatory and worsen gut symptoms in some women with endometriosis. Foods containing wheat or gluten may impair the gut lining and possibly affect the immune system, which could have an impact on endometriosis symptoms in susceptible women.

Dairy: While many studies actually suggest that high dairy intake decreases pain and endometriosis symptoms, many of our patients find it upsets the gut. Desi finds that many of her pelvic pain patients may have cow's dairy issues and so would recommend a trial removing cow's dairy if symptoms still persist after increasing fibre and reducing saturated fat and sugar. She finds that very few women have any adverse effects with goat and sheep cheese and yoghurt products so they may be suitable even if you find that cow's dairy exacerbates symptoms.

Desi also finds that many women are able to reintroduce small amounts of yoghurt and things like small amounts of sourdough bread after implementation of a Mediterranean diet once their gut health is in better shape.

If you can, try to buy organic fruit and vegetables and pasture-fed and/or organic animal products. Pesticides and other chemicals in food have been positively associated with endometriosis symptoms by interfering with hormonal pathways and contributing to inflammation.

Most of all trust and listen to your body and what feels right for you.

A NOTE ON HIGHLY RESTRICTIVE DIETS

Young women diagnosed with IBS, or endometriosis or who have pelvic pain and gut issues, often end up on restrictive diets such as low-FODMAP, gluten- or dairy-free diets. In most cases these young women have some degree of autonomic nervous system dysregulation, which is usually the prime reason for their pain and/or gastrointestinal symptoms.

Restricting their diet may help with symptoms initially, but given they're often already anxious and hypervigilant, it can make things worse by reinforcing hypervigilant behaviour without addressing the overall heightened nervous system. I've seen many young women who may have unresolved trauma, chronic stress and perfectionistic and anxious personalities go down this pathway of restricted eating, some of them ending up with an eating disorder.

I think that whole food groups should only be restricted under the guidance of a trauma-informed dietician who is aware of the risks of worsening or creating disordered eating. Modern science tells us that IBS is a disorder of the gut–brain axis – in other words of the vagus nerve, which is the prime messenger between our brain and our gut. While restrictive diets such as a low-FODMAP diet can be helpful in identifying certain dietary triggers, as dietician Desi Carlos says, they should never be a long-term solution and can do more harm than good in women with trauma and who may be experiencing restricted eating patterns.

The latest research on IBS tells us that mind–body treatments such as gut hypnotherapy are extremely effective at reducing gastrointestinal symptoms, with multiple good-quality studies showing a 70–80 per cent improvement in symptoms in people with IBS. Gut-directed hypnotherapy is one method of reprogramming the autonomic nervous system, by working on the vagus nerve to help people find their way out of fight, flight or freeze and into the ventral vagal state of rest and digest.

Supplements and botanical medicines

As part of a holistic treatment approach, some women may find certain supplements beneficial. Large studies looking at the effectiveness of supplements are limited, but some that show promise include:

- **curcumin (turmeric)**, which in endometriosis lesions accelerates healthy cell death, suppresses local production of oestrogen and inhibits formation of new blood vessels as well as blocking the effects of toll-like receptors. The usual dose is 1000 milligrams twice daily.
- **zinc**, which repairs intestinal permeability to help normalise immune function, is anti-inflammatory and helps to relieve pain. The usual dose is 30 milligrams a day taken with food.
- **NAC** (N-acetyl cysteine amino acid), an antioxidant and immune regulator that can help reduce inflammation and pain. In a very small 2013 study of 92 women, 47 took 600 milligrams of NAC three times a day for three months and 45 took a placebo. Of those who took NAC, 24 women (i.e. half) cancelled their scheduled laparoscopy due to a decrease in symptoms or because they had become pregnant, compared with one woman in the placebo group.
- **magnesium**, taken daily or with periods, it has been shown in some studies to be more effective than a placebo at improving period pain. It works as an anti-prostaglandin to reduce inflammation. The usual dose is 300 milligrams at night

throughout the cycle and/or 300–600 milligrams during the period. I usually recommend magnesium glycinate because magnesium citrate can cause loose stools in some women.

- **fish oil (omega-3)**, which reduces prostaglandin synthesis and thus inflammation. The suggested dose is 1000 milligrams daily.
- **vitamin D**, several studies have shown if a blood test reveals low vitamin D levels, vitamin D supplements may improve period pain by reducing prostaglandin synthesis.
- **probiotics**, which are helpful in restoring a healthy gut biome and reducing gut symptoms and pelvic pain.

My go-to supplement prescription

My go-to prescription for initial period pain if education, unwinding the nervous system, reducing stress, a healthy diet and simple analgesics are not working is:

- magnesium, 300 milligrams at night
- zinc, 30 milligrams a day
- omega-3 as fish oil, 1000 milligrams daily
- vitamin D if low, dose dependent on levels found in a blood test
- curcumin, 1000 milligrams daily or twice a day with periods
- ginger root capsules, 500 milligrams three times a day with periods.

I may consider adding the other supplements listed above if necessary, but all the supplements in the world won't help if you don't address the effects of stress hormones and nervous system dysregulation or if you're trying to outrun a poor diet.

Lifestyle

There's no direct evidence that lifestyle changes help women with endometriosis (because minimal studies have been done), but they make a huge difference to our patients every day. We know that having a healthy lifestyle helps our nervous system feel safe and also promotes a healthy immune system to reduce inflammation.

What to do

Particularly important parts of the lifestyle prescription to set you up for a healthy period are:

- **physical activity**. I recommend moving your body every day in a way that feels good to you. Tuning in to your body as its physiology changes throughout the menstrual cycle and adjusting the type of exercise is important. It's okay to slow down during your menstrual phase, but some form of gentle movement always helps decrease inflammation, release tight muscles and increase pain-reducing endorphins.
- **good sleep**. Getting seven to eight hours of sleep a night is incredibly important for immune function. It's also known to decrease cortisol and insulin, which results in lower inflammation and lower pain. This means going to bed mostly around the same time every night, minimising the use of screens close to bedtime and even introducing a nightly bedtime routine that allows you to wind down – stopping work or study a few hours before bed; minimising bright lights and going screen-free; having a bath or shower; and doing some gentle yoga, stretches, meditation or breath work before your head hits the pillow. This all helps promote the release of melatonin – which we need to help us feel sleepy and acts as an antioxidant in the body. Creating a wind-down practice also reduces cortisol so that you can fall into an easeful sleep where inflammation is low and the body can rest and repair.
- **avoiding endocrine-disrupting chemicals**. Chemicals such as phthalates, dioxins and PCBs could potentially have an impact on the growth of endometriosis. They are found in some plastics, synthetic fragrances, cosmetics and personal care products (including some pads and tampons), and cleaning products. They can mimic oestrogen in the body, and in rat studies have been associated with increased endometriosis growth. Try to minimise your use of plastics; choose natural products and

eat organic food when possible. You might also want to use organic pads or tampons or switch to period underwear or a menstrual cup. Minimising exposure to the thousands of chemicals that saturate modern life is, of course, optimal for human health in general. They are also implicated in increased rates of obesity, type 2 diabetes, early puberty, PCOS and male infertility.

- **living cyclically.** Try making room in your life for your body to rest when you have your period. The last part of this book will show you how it's possible to nurture your body throughout your whole cycle to set yourself up for an easeful period.

- **stress management and relaxation.** Chronically elevated cortisol can alter the gut microbiome, impair the gut lining, increase immune dysregulation and worsen other gut symptoms. Chronic stress increases the production of inflammatory cytokines and pelvic floor tension, and primes pain pathways to learn chronic pain. Learning how to spend more time in our parasympathetic nervous system state is the key (see Chapter 12).

- **hormonal drugs.** These include the combined oral contraceptive Pill, progestin-only pills such as Visanne or Slinda, and the progestin-containing IUDs – Mirena and Kyleena (see Chapter 4). For some women, hormonal drugs can be part of a holistic prescription for pelvic pain. The pills work by suppressing the growth of the uterus lining and/or suppressing ovulation and effectively turning off the cycle. This enables women to stay on continuous hormone pills and 'skip' their periods. The hormonal IUDs don't routinely suppress ovulation but do suppress the growth of the uterine lining and usually reduce or stop bleeding. Decreasing the amount of bleeding reduces the release of prostaglandins associated with a period, and also reduces the flow of menstrual blood into the pelvis and irritation from prostaglandins there. As long as you understand the potential side effects of these options (see Chapter 4), they can be part of the recipe to reduce inflammation and pain.

These changes on their own may not be enough

While a healthy diet, supplements, herbal treatments, reducing environmental toxins and even taking hormonal drugs have their place and can often make a big difference to women suffering with pelvic pain, the crux of the matter is that nothing will work if you don't feel safe in your body. You can be eating the 'cleanest' diet, have had the best excisional surgery, be on all the supplements, or have total menstrual suppression, but if you still don't feel safe – you have fear, unprocessed trauma or ongoing stress – and you are spending much of your time in fight, flight or freeze, there's a good chance your pain will persist.

If you have painful periods and find that your pain is still severe, debilitating or persistent after trying these simple strategies, something is wrong and you shouldn't ignore it. Persistent pain is always a sign that something is amiss, so you need to listen to it and get to the root of what it's trying to tell you. If you've been diagnosed with endometriosis and still have pain, there's usually far more to it than a laparoscopy can discover or treat.

Chapter summary

- The first step to healing period pain is menstrual cycle education to help demystify what's happening in the body and reduce fear.
- Making time for your period in your life, listening to your body and giving it what it needs, are important for reducing stress that can increase pain.
- A healthy wholefood diet reduces inflammation and supports gut and microbiome health.
- A bespoke period pain prescription may include ibuprofen/ Ponstan, tranexamic acid (for heavy periods), other anti-inflammatory herbs and supplements, and discussion about hormonal therapies.
- You should feel you have lots of options, information and the support to make the choices that feel right for you.

11

A holistic framework for treating persistent pelvic pain

If you have severe or persistent pain that hasn't responded to the simple strategies set out in the previous chapter, or you've been diagnosed with endometriosis and find yourself living with debilitating pain or symptoms despite the standard treatments, this chapter is for you. The women I see have rarely tried the simple things beforehand. Often they are already on the Pill at a minimum and, apart from learning to be worried about endometriosis, have been given no understanding about the contributors to pain and the link between the environment, subsequent underlying general health and their experience with their periods.

A recent survey of gynaecologists in the UK showed that 45 per cent of them felt uncomfortable managing chronic pelvic pain and many women with chronic pain are unsatisfied with their care. In women diagnosed with endometriosis (only some of whom will have chronic pain) many will have no relief from pain at all after surgery and of those that do, more than half will have a recurrence of pain, while 30–50 per cent of women who have had a laparoscopy to investigate pain will have no pathology found.

Visiting a gynaecologist

If you've tried the simple strategies in Chapter 10, the next step is to see a GP or gynaecologist who can look for deep endometriosis by doing a high-resolution transvaginal ultrasound if you're sexually active or a pelvic MRI if you're not. I never do a diagnostic laparoscopy without first doing a good-quality ultrasound or MRI. In recent years, these imaging techniques have become much more sensitive at detecting more significant types of endometriosis, and ultrasound remains the gold standard for ruling out any other pelvic pathology that could cause pain.

Imaging tests for endometriosis

Remember, all endometriosis isn't the same. The most 'severe' (although not necessarily correlated with pain), are usually ovarian endometriosis (endometriomas) and deep-infiltrating endometriosis, while the vast majority (80 per cent) of endometriosis found at laparoscopy is superficial and very likely a by-product of normal menstruation. Transvaginal pelvic ultrasound or MRI in expert hands has more than 90 per cent sensitivity for deep and ovarian endometriosis. If your scan is normal with no evidence of endometriosis, ovarian cysts, adhesions or any other pathology, then if there is any endometriosis at all it is likely to be superficial. This is reassuring.

If your scan does show some deep endometriosis and you have pain, the endometriosis may be contributing to your pain – but if your pain is chronic, we almost certainly need to pay attention to other parts of the puzzle as well.

If your specialist recommends surgery

The presence of endometriosis on a good-quality imaging study does not necessarily mean you need surgery, but if you do opt for surgery, ensure you choose a surgeon who specialises in excisional endometriosis surgery. Remember, though, that surgery is not benign, and not only that it might not improve pain but it could make pain worse. It's important to make sure you talk through the possible risks with your doctor, that your doctor takes into account your preferences, and that you talk through the non-surgical and non-hormonal options.

If your doctor says surgery is the only option and recommends repeat surgeries when your pain returns, I would strongly recommend seeking a second opinion. As evidenced by the number of women I see in my office still in pain after multiple operations, repeat surgery is often not a sustainable or effective solution as it doesn't address the root of chronic pain. It's as simple as that.

QUESTIONS TO ASK YOUR GYNAECOLOGIST BEFORE DECIDING ON SURGERY FOR PELVIC PAIN

1. What are the chances of my pain improving after laparoscopy and what is the chance that my pain will recur after surgery?
2. What are the risks of surgery?
3. Are you an experienced endometriosis surgeon?
4. What happens if I don't have surgery?
5. What are the other potential causes for my pain?
6. What alternative therapies might improve my pain?

If you do decide to have an initial surgery and you have chronic pain, make sure your doctor is addressing your nervous system, brain, pelvic floor and gut at the same time. As we have seen, simply treating the pelvis will not, in most cases, have long-lasting benefits. You may decide, like many of my patients, to work on addressing the other factors first and resort to surgery only if things aren't improving. The key thing to remember is that you do have options and that the presence of endometriosis on a scan could be relevant but could be a bit player in your pain story.

As a rule, if a woman with pelvic pain has a normal pelvic ultrasound, before doing a laparoscopy I would usually spend at least six months working on reducing inflammation, potentially reducing the inflammation of menstruation with hormones, relaxing the pelvic floor and working on increasing safety and stability in the body with nervous-system training. In my experience, after complete pain education and working on all these factors, only a small number of my patients go on to laparoscopy because their pain is significantly improved and their positive connection to their bodies is much deeper.

When I do talk about surgery, it's as just one part of a comprehensive menu of treatment options and after I've taken a thorough history to flesh out that patient's specific underlying causes of pain. I also tell my patients about the studies on pain and surgery and the paradox of pain with endometriosis. In simple terms, I provide them with all the information about what could be causing their pain, and all the science to date about the pros and cons of each treatment option. When I do this, I find that most women with pain actually choose conservative treatment over surgery and go on to do really well. Explanation of pain, giving options and tools to women to help themselves reduces their fear and gives them back power and autonomy. This alone helps to bring them back into their window of tolerance rather than a stress or survival state.

I should emphasise that the longer pain goes untreated, the more likely it is to persist, so I feel that the earlier pain is recognised, investigated and addressed the better. To me, however, this does not mean an early operation.

When I was a younger doctor I would, as I was taught, tend to recommend laparoscopy to anyone who had hadn't improved after three months of hormonal medications or simple non-steroidal anti-inflammatories. I would remove any endometriosis *and* also work on diet, pelvic floor and pain pathways, and my patients would usually do very well. Later I came to question whether it was the laparoscopy making them well or all the other things, and if it was all the other things, whether it wouldn't make more sense to address them and then go on to surgery if things didn't improve. I found that by doing this, in effect turning the pain iceberg upside down and starting with the big-picture things first – trauma, the nervous system, pain pathways, pelvic floor, the immune system and inflammation – my patients still got better and most didn't need surgery at all. And if they did, they were more likely to do better because all of the pathways to pain were being addressed, not just the tip of the iceberg.

Digging to the roots of chronic pelvic pain

If you have ongoing or severe period and/or pelvic pain, you *have* to look beyond the pelvis and dig down to the roots. Here you might find:

- a dysregulated autonomic nervous system due to trauma and/or chronic stress
- gut microbiome disturbance and/or intestinal hyperpermeability, immune dysfunction and increased inflammation. This disturbance can be due to stress and/or trauma or poor diet and exposure to endocrine-disrupting chemicals
- pelvic floor muscle tension – contraction and immobilisation
- upregulation of pain pathways and of the part of the brain that processes pain – pain system hypersensitivity (see Chapter 7)
- negative cultural and social attitudes to periods and women's bodies
- fear about endometriosis.

CASE STUDY: MELINDA

Melinda was 16 when she came to see me a few years ago. She had painful periods but also evidence of chronic pain, which occurred on most days. We had a huge talk about all the factors involved, including her dialled-up nervous system and pelvic floor tightness. Melinda was happy to try some amitriptyline (Endep) – to decrease the sensitivity of her pain pathways – and a Mirena IUD to suppress bleeding, but she still wanted a laparoscopy even after learning that the procedure could diagnose endometriosis and remove lesions but might not help with pain.

At laparoscopy she had mild (grade 1) endometriosis – the superficial, likely physiological kind. I excised it completely and inserted her Mirena at the same time. Six weeks later she was feeling better and her periods had stopped. She then didn't come back to see me for a few years. When I saw her again she was 18 and about to start university. She had increased pain on the left side and a pelvic ultrasound had revealed a left ovarian 'cyst'. Her GP's referral said: 'Melinda is concerned that her endometriosis is growing back.'

When I scanned Melinda she had a normal left ovary and a dominant follicle on the right ovary – exactly the same size as the previous scan had described the left ovarian cyst. She had a very tight pelvic floor but no pain around the left or right ovary or uterus. When I listened to what else was happening in her life, Melinda told me that she'd been having heightened anxiety lately in relation to the stress of Year 12 exams and starting uni. She had also not got around to seeing the pelvic floor physiotherapist and had gone off her Endep around six months earlier. She recognised that despite the fact she wasn't having any bleeding with the Mirena, her pain was worse when her anxiety was worse. She also noted that while her pain was more generalised before, it had become more left-sided after her GP told her she had a cyst there.

I explained to Melinda that the cysts were normal follicles and were evidence that her ovaries were functioning just the way they are supposed to. There was no evidence of anything pathological at all in her pelvis. There was still evidence, though, that she was holding all her tension in an overactive pelvic floor, and that she had upregulated pain pathways and a dysregulated autonomic nervous system.

She told me that she often didn't feel hungry, was experiencing more constipation and was having trouble sleeping – all signs of a nervous system in a survival state. Our plan was for her to begin seeing our pelvic floor physiotherapist and also our embodiment coach, Claire Stephensen, to help with strategies to calm her nervous system and reduce anxiety. Instead of the Endep, she started taking duloxetine – which helps to dial down pain pathways but also helps with anxiety. I assured Melinda that she didn't need more surgery, but that the recurrence of her pain was telling her something important about her nervous system that was important for her to address. Doing so would reduce her pain and inflammation, and help reverse the effects that chronic nervous system dysregulation can have on the body over time.

I caught up with Melinda 6 months later and asked her how her pain was. She said: 'Gone. After seeing Brooke, when the pain comes now, I know how to make it go away almost immediately.' Melinda told me that her anxiety had also gone after she made the decision to listen to what that feeling was trying to tell her, rather than push it away. Through working with Claire, Melinda realised that she didn't want to continue with the uni course she was enrolled in and wanted to go down a different path instead. She was loving learning to feel her feelings, including her physical sensations, in that grounded and safe part of her nervous system, rather than simply trying to push them away.

Melinda learnt that when she became aware enough to lean into what she was feeling, rather than going into protection or numbing mode, she could hear the wisdom of her body and was able to give her body what it needed to feel safe. Melinda was relaxed, happy, no longer in pain and no longer described herself as feeling anxious or depressed. The power of whole-person treatment is that, in addressing the roots, you don't just fix one symptom; you give a person the tools to know and help themselves, which has ripple effects into not only the patient's life but the lives of those around them.

The pain spiral

The factors listed above exist in the context of menstruation being a naturally inflammatory process where inflammatory prostaglandins are produced to enable the uterine lining to shed, and where the muscular wall contracts, sometimes producing cramps. All of these contributors to severe or persistent pain either amplify inflammation and hence pain, or amplify the perception of pain due to a dysregulated nervous system state that in turn creates more inflammation and pain in a vicious cycle.

By looking at this pain spiral you can see that an increased inflammatory state with or without endometriosis is potentially a downstream effect of autonomic nervous system dysregulation due to the feeling of an unsafe environment. Many factors can increase the pain and inflammation associated with periods, and many others can prime our nervous system to amplify and continue to drive this pain. Endometriosis is one factor out of many, and in many cases is likely to be an effect rather than the sole cause, while in many others it's an incidental finding. All of the factors in the pain spiral can affect each other and they can all cause pain.

When women have been told the story that endometriosis is the only thing that causes pain and that treatment starts and ends with surgery, they are disillusioned when they don't feel better after surgical excision. Many women with persistent pain are still at a loss as to just what is contributing to their ongoing symptoms. You haven't failed. You usually don't need more surgery. You just need to know all the things that could contribute and work out which ones apply to you.

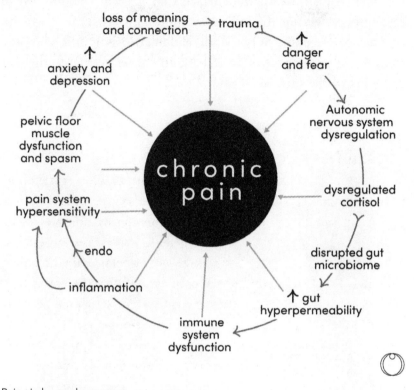

Pain circle graph. SOURCE: Vera Women's Wellness.

Once you can name your personal contributing factors and connect the dots, you can start addressing each part of the puzzle – just like peeling away the layers of an onion. The overarching layer is the nervous system – nothing works until you start feeling safe in your body and your environment. Chronic pain is a systemic issue and we need to start looking at both the unconscious autonomic nervous system that governs our bodily functions and our pain pathway system, which can be turned up or down depending on the state of safety in our autonomic nervous system. If you have chronic pain and your health practitioner is not talking about these overarching issues, you need to find someone else who will help you get to the root of the problem and achieve true healing.

The pain iceberg

Looking at the contributors to chronic pelvic pain, there's clearly so much lying beneath the surface that it seems obvious we're setting ourselves up for failure by thinking that surgery will fix chronic pelvic pain. Surgery for endometriosis is like chipping away at the upper part of an iceberg and never getting to the real cause below the surface.

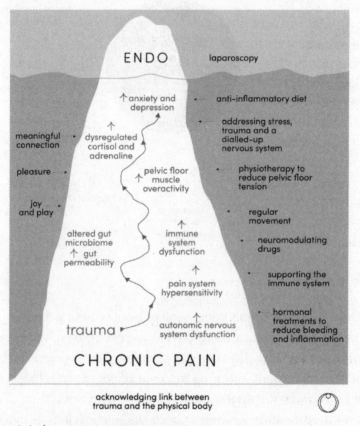

Endo pain iceberg. SOURCE: Vera Women's Wellness.

How we heal chronic pelvic pain

The most important thing in the healing journey is time and space for your story to be told, for you to feel listened to without judgement and to feel like your doctor cares about you first and foremost and about helping you to live the life you want. You want to leave the doctor's office feeling heard, that someone is on your side and that you have a plan.

With or without a history of endometriosis, here's how we would treat each part of the iceberg on page 170.

For pain system hypersensitivity

Our approach at Vera Women's Wellness would generally include:

- pain education (see Part 1)
- brain retraining to reduce fear (see Chapter 14)
- neuromodulating drugs, such as amitriptyline (Endep), nortriptyline or duloxetine
- trial of low-dose naltrexone (LDN) which decreases neuro-inflammation through blocking TLR4 and increasing the brain's production of natural endorphins.

Neuromodulating drugs can be useful at turning down the sensitivity of the nervous system by blocking the action of TLR4 and, in the case of duloxetine, also help with anxiety. They can have side effects such as drowsiness, dry mouth or eyes, but generally only with larger doses.

These drugs can be useful for a short time while you work on techniques for downregulating your pain pathways and receive physiotherapy, but can also be continued long-term. Most of my patients usually come off them after six months to a year. Small doses of amitriptyline can also be used for a pain flare.

For a dysregulated autonomic nervous system

Our approach would generally encompass:

- education on the autonomic nervous system and polyvagal theory (see Chapter 8)
- therapy for working through trauma (see Chapter 13)
- learning techniques for returning to a place of safety in the nervous system (see Chapter 12).

For pelvic floor tension

Pelvic floor physiotherapy (see Chapter 15) is the cornerstone of our therapy for chronic pelvic pain. Sometimes if the pelvic floor is really wound up and not responding to at least three months of physiotherapy, Botox can be injected into the muscles of the pelvic floor. This works just like Botox for crow's feet – by paralysing the muscles and releasing muscle tension. The available evidence shows it can have significant effects in reducing pain at up to six months after treatment. It's not a magic bullet though. The aim is to relax your pelvic floor enough for you to be able to engage successfully in physiotherapy. While this is a tool in my toolbox, I usually find that most women do incredibly well with a good physiotherapist who can teach them how to connect to their pelvic floor themselves and reach a state of relaxation in their own body.

Sometimes a muscle relaxant such as Valium as a suppository can be really helpful for pain flares if the pelvic floor is really wound up.

For gut health

Our techniques could include:

- focusing attention on finding safety in the nervous system (see Chapter 12), including using apps such as Nerva or a trauma-informed dietician to engage the vagus nerve and set the scene for healthy digestion
- a Mediterranean anti-inflammatory diet (see Chapter 10).

For reducing inflammation

In this instance we would focus on things such as:

- hormone medications (see Chapter 4)
- supplements, herbs such as ginger root and non-steroidal anti-inflammatories such as ibuprofen and paracetamol (see Chapter 10).

CASE STUDY: DANA

Dana was 32 when she came to see me. She had been diagnosed with endometriosis at laparoscopy in her early twenties and had it excised. She and her ex-girlfriend shared a little boy who had been carried by her ex-partner. Dana commented that because of her history of endometriosis, the fertility specialist had recommended that she not carry the baby.

She was single when she came to see me and her main goals were 'to get rid of period pain' and have a plan for her endometriosis. Although each month she suffered two days of severe period pain, she also had significant abdominal pain, bloating and irritable bowel symptoms. She often tended towards constipation and found that she was very sensitive to FODMAP foods, particularly onion and garlic. She was hyperaware of any gas or bloating sensation. Dana was particularly worried because she felt sharp pain on passing a motion – a bit like a hot poker in her bottom. This sensation was always more intense around ovulation and periods. She also noted sharp pain during and after high-intensity interval training and other strenuous activities.

She was concerned about a recurrence of her endometriosis, particularly because of her bowel symptoms and what she had read about the possibility of bowel or recto-vaginal endometriosis. From what she had read and her experience so far, she felt that surgery was probably the next step in treating her symptoms.

Dana had quite a bit of stress in her life, especially since her acrimonious relationship breakdown and with the pressures of being a single mum. She told me she had been sexually assaulted as a teenager. She had suffered from anxiety since her teenage years.

When I examined Dana, her pelvic ultrasound was normal with no signs of deep-infiltrating endometriosis. She had no pain around her cervix or ovaries. Her pelvic floor examination revealed tight pelvic floor muscles and tenderness that could reproduce the pain sensation she felt during her period.

Although I hadn't done a laparoscopy, and so couldn't completely rule out that some of her pain might have been related to potential superficial endometriosis, Dana had definite evidence of an overactive pelvic floor, with constricted and tight muscles around her vagina and anus. She also had ongoing gastrointestinal pain and other symptoms related to poor digestion, despite a highly restrictive diet.

When we put it all together, it was obvious that prior trauma and the subsequent upregulation of Dana's nervous system to be on high alert for danger – both in the outside world and within her body – were probably contributing to her symptoms. Before even considering whether an endometriosis diagnosis was relevant, it was clear to me that the overarching theme in Dana's life of persistent stress and a dysregulated autonomic nervous system was causing some if not all of her troubling symptoms. I explained the idea of polyvagal theory and how being stuck in fight, flight and freeze impacts every system in our body. Dana could see how all of this made sense in theory and was open to exploring how taking a step back from a lesion-focused approach and taking a big-picture view of the body could help.

I gave Dana the facts about what surgery to remove endometriosis can and can't achieve, and allowed her to make her own decision about whether she thought it was the right option for her. She decided to try the whole-body and nervous system approach for the next few months before revisiting the idea of surgery.

This meant that Dana would see Brooke for pelvic floor relaxation and nervous system down-training; and dietician, Elissa, to focus on her gut health. But this time, rather than taking more out of an already restricted diet, Elissa talked Dana through how her nervous system could be affecting her gastrointestinal symptoms. She even enrolled in a yoga course with an emphasis on calming the vagus nerve to improve pain and the effects of stress on the body.

When I saw Dana three months later, she was blown away by the changes she had already experienced in her body. She had been practising breathing exercises and pelvic floor stretches daily, and engaging in an online gut hypnotherapy course for her IBS symptoms in addition to working one on one with Brooke and Elissa. Dana's bloating and abdominal pain had reduced significantly, her bowel movements had become regulated, and her pain associated with passing a bowel motion and with her periods had become almost non-existent. She had some discomfort with periods but didn't need to take anything more than ginger and magnesium for cramps. She was even able to reintroduce some of the high-FODMAP foods such as onion and garlic that she had been unable to tolerate before.

Dana felt that through receiving accurate education about endometriosis and other causes of pelvic pain and addressing her dialled-up nervous system, her fear of endometriosis as a scary disease had reduced, along with her pain and symptoms. She also felt that her overall health was improved and that the whole-body and nervous system approach wasn't just a band-aid for a symptom. Dana was grateful for having been shown a different way that allowed her to take control of her own body and her own healing in a supported manner. She was confident that if she had not stumbled across our clinic and our way of seeing things, she would probably have had surgery and not addressed the underlying problems.

Diving right to the root of your pain

Understanding all the factors that lie at the root of pelvic pain can be life-changing for women because it's validation. Validation that of course there *is* something wrong. It isn't all in our heads. We haven't tried everything and failed. We just haven't been shown what's beneath the surface of our pain. It's not our failure. No one has listened or looked into the depths of where most of the problems lie. Not just within our bodies, but also within our environment and the wider social network that is unsafe for a female body. Even if you think you have had the perfect life with no trauma – the trauma of living in a world that isn't made for you is real. If you suffer with chronic pelvic pain you have likely felt the trauma of dealing with a medical system where you felt lost, dismissed or simply like you had no power over your 'broken body'. This layers trauma upon trauma and continues to change your nervous system, exacerbating pain and making you even more disconnected from your body. We can't tackle or address something until we can name it and see it. Understanding how pain develops and persists is therapeutic in itself.

So let's go there. Let's take that deep dive and look at what *your* pain is a symptom of – what lies beneath the surface. Unless we do that, we can never get to the true root of the problem. I know this might feel confronting, scary or even triggering. For many women there are very good reasons why traumas remain buried and why they may be afraid to acknowledge or let go of maladaptive coping strategies – it's a survival mechanism after all. Sometimes locking our traumas away is the only way we can carry on, as some experiences can be too painful or frightening to feel fully.

For all women with chronic pain, nervous system dysregulation lies at the base of the pain iceberg and we can't continue to ignore it. For this reason, after ruling out significant anatomical pathology, the most important beginning your doctor could make is simply allowing time and space for them to truly hear your whole story. This not only gives you the chance to deal with the problem at its foundation, but provides a space where you can be truly seen and heard, where you can begin to dig down to expose the roots of your pain story. Down to the hidden, dark places where trauma resides in the body.

The principles of trauma therapy

These are threefold:

1. Finding safety and stability.
2. Exploring your pain story to help explain why your body has become stuck.
3. Integration – finding meaning and connection, joy and pleasure.

We will cover points 1 and 2 in the remaining chapters of Part 2, and move on to point 3 in Part 3 of the book.

Before we dig down to the roots of your personal story, I want to ensure that you know how to bring your nervous system to a point where it feels a degree of safety. Some questions about your past might trigger feelings of danger or anxiety within your body, so it's so important to be able to begin only when your nervous system feels safe and stabilised. This is the first step in healing chronic pain and nervous system dysregulation.

Chapter summary

- Treatment for chronic pelvic pain is multi-layered and considers the whole person, not just a lesion.
- If you have pain system hypersensitivity, treatment should be focused on the nervous system.
- If you have evidence of severe endometriosis on imaging and opt for surgery, ensure you are still addressing all of the factors at the bottom of the iceberg. Otherwise it is more likely your pain will persist.
- If you opt for surgery make sure your surgeon is well-trained in endometriosis surgery.

12

Finding safety and stability in your nervous system

It's safe to say that most, if not all, people who experience chronic pain are stuck in a state of nervous system dysregulation – whether or not they have experienced a traumatic childhood or a past traumatic experience. Understanding how to regulate your nervous system is therefore hugely important if you have chronic pain. Before we dig down into the roots of the experiences that could have shaped your nervous system, in this chapter I provide some tools that will allow you to come back to safety in your nervous system, especially if you feel triggered as you read the next chapter of this book.

Unresolved trauma and/or chronic stress lead to being stuck in fight, flight or freeze. By definition, we need to be in a state of fear to become stuck in these states. Fear always perpetuates chronic pain. As we saw in Chapter 7, having a dysregulated nervous system leads to either prolonged sympathetic activation (fight or flight) or a prolonged dorsal vagal state (freeze). These states represent either anxiety and hypervigilance – amplification of all senses inside in the body – or total disconnection from the body. Our primal or caveperson brain can't distinguish a real threat to our lives, such as a gun pointing at our head, starvation or a lion chasing us, from perceived threats that also cause a rise in adrenaline and cortisol, such as relationship stress, work or school pressures, or not feeling accepted and safe enough to be our authentic selves. This old operating system is hardwired into us. It hasn't been updated for our modern lives in Western society, where high levels of perceived stress are the norm. This represents a form of biological–evolutionary mismatch, where the biological features that helped us survive in a very different environment thousands of years ago are no longer a survival advantage when persistently activated under the high-stress environment we find ourselves in today.

Fight, flight, freeze and pain

Sympathetic activation (fight or flight) leads to increased hyper-vigilance, which means our nervous system – including our pain pathway system – becomes turned up to 10/10 on the sensitivity scale. Our systems become highly attuned to detect danger in our environment. Our brain notices any sensation as more intense, so that potentially painful stimuli become debilitating – rather than a mild ache, and even neutral body sensations such as pressure, touch or internal digestion sensations become painful. Safe stimuli or situations are often misinterpreted as dangerous and trigger our body into even further activation of our fight, flight or freeze states. This happens both from sensations within the body (interoception) and from our external environment (neuroception). It may make us more likely to behave defensively to people in our life, which makes real connection and building and keeping healthy relationships difficult.

Elevated adrenaline and cortisol also slow digestion, which can lead to bloating, IBS, dysbiosis (gut microbiome imbalance) and leaky gut. This is because if the brain senses danger, the body goes into survival mode, where digestion is not a priority. This all contributes to excess inflammation and immune system dysfunction. A chronically dysregulated nervous system is associated with higher release of inflammatory chemicals. Our muscles, including those in our pelvic floor, become tight and contracted as a protective mechanism.

Often with chronic pain, we stop moving for fear that movement will lead to more pain; this immobilisation (which is often seen in dorsal vagal or freeze states) starts as a way to protect us from pain, but if we're not moving, our brain interprets that to mean movement is dangerous and hence the cause of pain is dangerous and something to fear. Fear will always produce more pain in the brain.

The freeze state might also leave you more disconnected from your body, with poor digestion and chronic fatigue symptoms. If your level of stress or trauma has been so overwhelming that you find yourself in freeze, your brain thinks it's too dangerous to move and use up resources, so your body may experience fatigue as a way to get you to stop and conserve energy. Both dysregulated states block your ability to experience a sense of pleasure or safety. They also make logical thinking more difficult, because prolonged stress often leads to reduced frontal lobe activity (the part of our brain that helps us think critically and plan). If you're stuck in these states, fear and a sense of danger will be subconsciously high whether you realise it or not, and pain is always generated by the brain because it's trying to protect you from danger.

If you experience chronic pelvic pain, it's highly likely that your nervous system is dysregulated. The first part of the process is to become aware not just of what's happening in your pelvis, but of how your body is feeling from a big-picture body–mind–spirit perspective.

Signs of a fight, flight or freeze state

You might be so used to feeling the dysregulated emotions and bodily sensations listed below that you have limited experience of what it feels like when your body is in its safe, balanced, ventral vagal state. With sympathetic activation, every bodily sensation is dialled up to 10/10 and you may feel like all your attention is fixated on those sensations, leaving you little room to notice your corresponding emotions. Or you if have unresolved trauma or persistent stress and are stuck in freeze because it doesn't feel safe to pay attention to the feelings in your body, you may have become so disconnected and disassociated from them that you simply have no awareness at all.

If you are stuck in or frequently triggered into a fight, flight or freeze state, these are the signs.

Fight or flight – sympathetic nervous system activation

The hypervigilance that results from sympathetic activation can lead to these emotions and physical symptoms.

Emotions

Anxiety, panic, fear, feeling 'wired', inability to rest, feeling angry, irritable or frustrated, rumination, constant worry, feeling overwhelmed.

Physical symptoms

Muscle tension leading to aches and pains, insomnia, being easily startled, shakiness, racing heart, bloating and digestive issues, autoimmune issues, headaches, grinding the teeth, increased inflammatory symptoms and altered immune function, cold fingers and toes.

Freeze – parasympathetic nervous system shutdown

These are the signs that indicate the parasympathetic nervous system has shut down.

Emotions

Depression, numbness, dissociation, shame, shutdown, hopelessness, going through the motions of life without actually living.

Physical symptoms

Exhaustion and chronic fatigue, weight gain due to a slowed metabolism and conservation of energy, immobilisation, impaired memory and concentration, digestive issues (often slowed digestion and constipation), reduced ability to make eye contact and relate to people.

Signs of a safe, regulated ventral vagal (parasympathetic) state

If your nervous system is regulated so that you feel safe and stabilised, this is how it feels.

Emotions

Feeling joyful, present, grounded, curious and open, compassionate and mindful.

Physical feelings

Optimal digestion and intestinal motility; feeling rested and able to relate and connect to yourself, others and the world around you; feeling relaxed and *safe*.

Exercise: Journaling on feelings of safety

Think back and see if you can remember a time where you felt safe, present and grounded. Journal on that memory and see if you can remember the sensations you felt in your body. Can you remember sights, smells, sounds, colours?

....

....

....

Understandably, if you have chronic pain and are either stuck in sympathetic activation and feeling overwhelmed or stuck in a freeze state of hopelessness, you might feel like this is all unchangeable.

You may not be able to do this exercise at all, or even be able to imagine a place where you could feel safe. But do believe me, the beauty of understanding our nervous system states and the nature of neuroplasticity means that it's very much changeable. Just as your nervous system has learned to stay in survival, it can also learn to find the pathway to safety. Read on and try the other exercises that come up.

Coming back into your window of tolerance

Having a healthy nervous system isn't about being in the safe ventral vagal state 100 per cent of the time. It's about becoming conscious enough to witness how you are feeling in your body at any given moment, checking in and reappraising if you're really in danger or whether you are in fact safe. If you can get to this place, you can use a whole host of tools to retrain your nervous system. This will help it remember you're safe in the present and not stuck in the past – and find its way back home to your parasympathetic state of safety, where both pain and fear are reduced.

A very useful way of thinking about fight, flight and freeze is viewing your safe ventral vagal state as your 'window of tolerance'. This is the sweet spot where you can handle stress and cope in healthy ways with the challenges of life without your nervous system hitting the panic button and either falling into freeze (parasympathetic collapse) or escalating into fight or flight (sympathetic activation).

When we're carrying around unprocessed trauma or dealing with high levels of current stress, including that of chronic pain, our fuse is short. We're triggered easily and often respond to a small stressor in a big way, with a tendency to overreact or sink into overload and paralysis. Our nervous system has not been updated with the memo that the danger was in the past and not in our present day, and so still responds like the original danger is present and works quickly to bring you into your survival states. From here you might notice that you feel out of control, you can't think logically, and fear, panic or dread take over. You might feel the bodily sensations of fight, flight or freeze. Learning to regulate your nervous system means recognising your bodily sensations and when you've moved outside your window of tolerance, then using both thinking and feeling strategies to return to safety in your body.

As a trauma-informed practitioner I understand how thoughts, behaviours and feelings can be triggered more easily when you're living in a traumatised body. The most important part of working with someone is to provide them with an anchor to safety and stability before we move on to discussing individual traumatic events. Without this safe place to come back to, there is a risk of retraumatisation, which is obviously the opposite of our aim to reduce fear and find safety in the body.

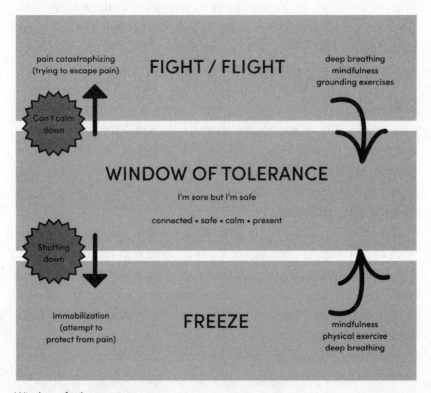

Window of tolerance

How to return to your window of tolerance

I want to teach you these simple strategies to bring you back to safety if you feel triggered in the pages to come and in the next chapter. Learning these tools is also vital for managing a pain flare that could potentially escalate you into a fight, flight or freeze state and make your pain worse.

Anytime you're feeling dysregulated or triggered, use these eleven practical ways to anchor back into safety and widen your window of tolerance: knowledge, mindfulness, breathing, tapping into your senses, journaling, listening to your favourite music, singing and chanting or even humming, touch, movement, immersing yourself in nature, and co-regulation. These are only some of the many ways you can begin to re-establish a sense of safety and stability in your nervous system. They're all free and accessible, and when practised regularly will help you immensely on your journey to know and care for yourself.

Here's how.

Knowledge

Simply understanding how your subconscious autonomic nervous system works can ground you because it provides a framework for understanding why your body might be responding a certain way. It allows you to feel compassion for yourself rather than self-blame or shame, so that your emotions don't spiral. It reduces fear, so that physical symptoms such as pain don't escalate. And it can help you recognise which state you're in so you can return to your window of tolerance.

Bringing yourself to conscious awareness is half the battle when addressing any problem, but simply by reading this book up to this point you're becoming a master in understanding and befriending your nervous system.

Mindfulness

This is the act of anchoring to the present moment. Deep breathing, aka breath practice or breath work (see below) and sense awareness are both examples, as is meditation. Reminding yourself that you're not in your past and using tools like breath awareness or a mantra to bring you back into the now helps your body to remember that you're safe in this moment without the need to relive past trauma or get stuck in fear. Pain often worsens when we remember past pain, fear future pain and start to engage in protective behaviours to avoid future pain. This is why being present in the moment is so important both in reducing physical pain and in bringing us out of past trauma into the safety of now.

Breathing

Taking deep belly breaths activates our vagus nerve, which helps us come back to that calm ventral vagal window. There are many different types of breath practice but all achieve the same goal – helping us feel safe. Remember, about 80 per cent of the fibres in the vagus nerve go from the body to the brain, so in breathing deeply we're telling our brain we're safe and bringing ourselves back to the present.

Some easy breathing exercises are taking a deep breath in for a count of four, then exhaling for a count of six or eight. The longer the exhale, the more we tap in to that calming vagal energy. My other favourite is box or square breathing, where you breathe in for a count of four, hold for a count of four, breathe out for four, hold for a count of four and then repeat.

Tapping into your senses

If you've been catapulted back into a survival state that belongs in the past, a great way to ground you back in your body in the here and now is to pay attention to your sensations. There are lots of ways to do this. One is to notice one thing you can see, one thing you can hear, one thing you can feel, one thing you can taste, and one thing you can smell. In this way you're utilising all your senses to bring you back into the now where you're safe.

Journaling

If you're stuck and find it difficult to identify, let alone feel, your feelings, you may benefit from putting your thoughts down on paper. Journaling is an evidence-based practice that can help you feel and then release difficult emotions. Even if no one sees it but you, the simple act of bringing awareness to your thoughts and feelings and expressing them has been shown to help with anxiety, depression and PTSD as well as physical stress symptoms including chronic pain.

Nicole Sachs is a psychotherapist and writer whose technique called Journal Speak uses journaling as therapy for people experiencing chronic pain. Her philosophy on the link between trauma, nervous system dysfunction and chronic pain aligns with mine, in that she believes 'chronic pain is but an entry point, inviting us to the precipice of truth which has been awaiting our acknowledgment'. This encapsulates the heart of the mind–body continuum and theorises that if we don't recognise and express our feelings about what happened to us and what we're going through, our body will express them through pain, discomfort and other physical symptoms. Nicole writes that 'once emotions are given a steam valve, the mind/body system is able to find equilibrium, moving from fight or flight to rest and repair and symptoms dissolve'.

You can journal each day by setting a timer for 20 minutes and free-writing whatever comes up, allowing it to bubble to the surface without feeling the need to judge it or second-guess yourself. What's there wants to be expressed, so let it. You can also do this when you feel yourself entering a dysregulated state. The act of being aware of your feelings and expressing them can help to bring you back into your window of tolerance.

The other thing I do with my clients if free-writing sounds too intimidating is to simply start with some basic prompts such as:

- Right now I feel . . .
- Today my body needs . . .
- How can I move my body in a way that feels good today?
- How can I experience pleasure in my body today even if I'm experiencing discomfort and pain?

Listening to your favourite music

Make a playlist of your favourite music. Or you might like to create several for different emotional states. One that's calming might help you out of hyperarousal (fight or flight), while one that's high-energy might help you out of hypoarousal (freeze or shutdown). Choose music that makes you feel safe or reminds you of a happy time. Music also activates our vagus nerve through our ears. Although this is intuitive, music therapy has been shown to reduce heart rate and blood pressure, and improve feelings of stress, anxiety and depression.

Singing and chanting or even humming

All three activate our vagus nerve and promote calm. If you think you can't sing – everyone can and it's for you only so it doesn't matter if you're hitting the right notes – try simply repeating the sound *hum* out loud and extending the *m* – so it sounds like *hummmmmm, hummmmmm, hummmmmmm*. There is even research showing that humming can improve heart rate variability, which is a measure of nervous system balance and regulation.

Touch

A hug from someone you feel safe with is incredibly regulating. If you don't have that person nearby, there are other ways you can use this sense to bring you into safety. For example, weighted blankets and acupressure mats can help activate pressure points on our skin that promote a sense of safety and security.

Movement

Moving our body is incredible for helping it discharge stress. Movement allows the adrenaline and cortisol to move through our body, and promotes the release of endorphins that help us feel better.

Think of a zebra that has fled a ravenous lion and has escaped. First the fight or flight system is activated, enabling the zebra to run fast and evade the lion's clutches. Once the threat of danger is over, the zebra might shake it out and five minutes later is happily grazing with the rest of the herd, having forgotten all about its close encounter with death. We humans, on the other hand, experience stress and trauma over and over again – and too often never learn how to complete the stress cycle and return to our regulated state.

Try dancing to your favourite songs, going for a run or a walk, doing some yoga or even actually literally shaking it off. Shaking therapy where you simply shake all parts of your body – hands, arms, shoulders, feet, legs, hips, chest and head – is used in trauma therapy and can be powerful at releasing feelings of stress, anxiety and anger. Even a burst of movement as short as 30 seconds can be beneficial. It's important to bring awareness to your emotions before and after movement, and to recognise that releasing trauma is always about allowing yourself to feel it so you can let it go. Movement brings our bodies out of shutdown, through sympathetic activation and back into our window of tolerance.

Immersing yourself in nature

Evidence abounds for the healing power of nature. In Japan, doctors prescribe forest bathing for stress, and studies show that spending time in nature helps to regulate our nervous system by reducing stress hormones, lowering blood pressure, reducing anxiety and nervous system arousal, and improving mood and immune system function. So find a tree, a patch of grass, an ocean, a creek or a mountain trail, and feel the way it allows your nervous system to drop into safety. We ourselves are nature, and grounding ourselves in it is deeply healing.

Co-regulation

This is when the loving presence of someone with a regulated nervous system can bring us back to safety in our body. It's as simple as the idea of a child being upset and being comforted by a caregiver. Having someone around who helps you feel safe is incredibly powerful. You can even co-regulate with a pet and by experiencing the oneness of nature (see above). Humans are wired for connection, and when we feel disconnected we become sick – physically and mentally. When we're out of our safe window it's hard to feel connected, but finding opportunities to co-regulate with safe, loving people and pets can help bring us back to our window of tolerance.

Exercise: Returning to safety

I want you to practise, right now, at least two of the eleven ways to find safety discussed above: knowledge, mindfulness, breathing, tapping into your senses, journaling, listening to your favourite music, singing and chanting or even humming, touch, movement, immersing yourself in nature, and co-regulation. Before we move to the next chapter, I want you to have tried a few of these practices and feel confident that they will help you return to your safe window. Before you start, become aware of how you feel. Write it down if it helps. Use these prompts:

- *How does your body feel?*
- *Describe your emotional state.*
- *Are you aware of your nervous system state? Are you hyperaroused (in fight or flight), hypoaroused (in freeze) or in your safe window? Check the signs listed on pages 180–82 if you're not sure how to tell.*

Engage in one of the activities, then answer these same questions again. Can you notice a shift?

Note: Initially try to practise these exercises when you're feeling relatively safe rather than when you're in the midst of an emotional crisis or a massive pain flare. Ideally you want to start practising when your pain is at a tolerable level. Sometimes trying when you're super dialled up can be counterproductive, especially when you're just learning these tools.

Read on in safety

Now that you have some tools to help you return to safety if you're triggered, we can move on to exploring your particular story. Please remember, if you've experienced severe trauma and feel afraid to acknowledge potentially upsetting memories, you don't have to read the next chapter. Alternatively, if you're worried that your trauma is too much to confront on your own, you might choose to do so with a safe person by your side – including your therapist, if you're working with one – who will be able to keep you anchored to that sense of safety and stability in the here and now. If you do omit the next chapter, though, I would encourage you to come back to it when you feel like you've restored your sense of stability. Acknowledging how trauma affects your body is crucial for moving forward, and learning how to return to a sense of safety in your body. Feeling safe is the key to rewiring your brain and nervous system and addressing your chronic pelvic pain.

Chapter summary

- Awareness is the first step in recognising whether you feel safe or in danger within your body.
- Noticing where you are in your nervous system means you can utilise tools to move back to safety if you are stuck in survival.
- There are many easy ways to bring yourself back to safety in your body – the place where your body works easefully and where pain is less likely.

13

Acknowledging trauma and stress in your life

As my friend Paula Hindle, an integrative women's health coach, physiotherapist, exercise physiologist and yoga teacher, so eloquently says: 'Every pelvis has a story. A big part of healing comes from listening to that story and allowing your body to be heard.' What is the story your pelvis is holding on to?

Even once you know that your chronic pain could be related to trauma, it can be difficult to bring it up in a medical setting for several reasons: fear of retraumatisation, the practitioner not having the required training, or the practitioner not even understanding that there is a very strong link between trauma and persistent pain. It's highly likely that a health practitioner has never asked you 'What happened to you?', 'Who was there for you?' or 'Tell me the story your body is trying to tell you through pain', only 'What's wrong with you?'

Recognising trauma

I've been a trauma-aware practitioner for many years now, so it's often incredibly obvious to me when a patient has experienced a capital-T, aka big-T trauma. When they've been through little-T traumas, the signs are more subtle. Capital-T traumas include horrific experiences such as sexual abuse, physical abuse, an acute accident, war, or death of a parent or family member early in life. These, particularly sexual trauma, are commonly intensely associated with pelvic pain. Often my patients have never told anyone about these traumas before, or have told someone they love only to be dismissed or not believed, which compounded the trauma. Little-T traumas are things like bullying at school, a relationship break-up, or divorce of parents.

Although many people are aware of describing trauma in this way, most experts no longer subscribe to this approach. This is because while one person may experience something objectively as very traumatic without becoming a traumatised person, another may experience something seemingly far less severe on a trauma scale but end up going through life stuck in a survival state. Anything that interferes with the crucial primary attachment between a child and a caregiver can have a huge effect on the nervous system. This might be due to a caregiver being unable to be present or actively attuned to their child's needs due to their own traumas or issues, or a physically absent parent.

Perhaps it's best to move beyond the very overused word *trauma* and simply think of it as the lasting emotional and physiological response that can result from living through a distressing event or series of events. Becoming traumatised can be the result of a single acute event or exposure to chronically stressful situations. Complex trauma describes ongoing and repeated trauma that usually begins in childhood and is often interpersonal in nature – meaning it often includes verbal, physical and sexual abuse, or neglect. This kind of complex trauma is often very difficult for people to identify because it's so pervasive. There is no one event, and many people internalise it as meaning they're bad or unlovable rather than seeing that they had no one to reliably care for their emotional needs.

In the most simple terms, trauma therapy for most people is recognising their body is not broken, they're not wrong, and that their clever, incredible brain and body have adapted to their environment. If we have experiences where we don't feel safe and we don't integrate or process those experiences, our nervous system can change to one of survival, altering our physiology and our health in our immediate and future life. Think of a tiny seed. If it's grown in nourishing soil replete with all the minerals it needs, just enough water and enough sunshine, a shoot will grow. If conditions remain optimal, it will become a tiny tree then grow into a straight tall tree – green and vibrant. If the soil isn't so good or there's not enough water or the sunlight is blocked, the tree adapts. It might grow crooked to try to find its way to the light or it might be stunted. It responds to its environment but it always has the potential to be that tall healthy tree.

For humans it's obviously more complex. The physical conditions of our environment are important, but so are our emotional conditions. Our emotional safety – our sense of belonging and being loved – is paramount. In this way, it's not only traumatic events that can change our physiology, but also the absence of love and acceptance. Humans are wired for connection and belonging. At a primal level, rejection is deeply distressing and traumatising for us. In ancient times being alone would often mean literal death. So when we feel that disconnection or rejection – even at an emotional level – it activates the same survival pathways as if we were actually thrown out of the tribe, and this changes our body and wires us for pain. After all, the same parts of the brain that process emotional pain process physical pain.

The many shades of developmental trauma
When you think of trauma or PTSD you may very likely think of huge and horrifying experiences like a natural disaster, a

serious car accident, sexual trauma or being in a war. But when you understand how the nervous system can change in response to incredibly common scenarios of early childhood, you can get a taste for just how pervasive and widespread the problem is. Developmental trauma has now been redefined to include any experience where you feel unseen, unheard or unsafe to express who you authentically are.

Many of the women I see may tell me straight off the bat that they had a 'normal' childhood with no traumatic events that they recognise. But incredibly often, these same women then recount being part of a family dynamic where they had incredibly high expectations placed on them, had to walk on eggshells around family members, lived with a chronically ill family member, had a parent who was obsessed with body size and weight, or moved school five times and always struggled to fit in. Many of these women would actually fit the diagnostic criteria for complex PTSD.

Some people say everything was fine but then recount that they were in a humidicrib for six weeks after they were born prematurely and separated from their mother or caregiver. Others may have had parents who divorced when they were too young to remember and so think it didn't affect them. The research reveals the contrary. Bruce Perry, a psychiatrist and one of the world's leading experts on childhood trauma and how it affects the brain, says that the earlier a child or infant experiences something traumatic – separation, neglect, abuse – the more severe the effects on their brain and nervous system.

The importance of healthy attachment cannot be overstated. At a recent workshop I attended, I heard Bessel van der Kolk say that 'attachment trumps trauma' and that while it's important to ask 'What happened to you?', it's even more important to ask 'Who was there for you?' He asserts that people are much more likely to thrive after an objectively traumatic event when they have someone to go to who loves and cares for them, but when no one is there for them the experience of trauma is far more likely to persist in the body and brain. The effects of a disrupted attachment are amplified if they occur early on in a child's life when their brain and nervous system are developing. An insecure attachment changes the wiring of the brain and pushes children into a fight, flight or freeze survival state, leading to all the changes in physiology we've already discussed.

When we think of how little support we provide parents in our society, we can see how far more frequently trauma begins in our homes, not on a battlefield. They are often left to parent by themselves without the support of the village they were meant to have, or they are suffering with postnatal depression or anxiety, or they are overwhelmed because both parents need to work full-time outside the home. The critical value of the child–caregiver relationship is summed up beautifully by Bessel van der Kolk, who says, 'The parent–child connection is the most powerful mental health intervention known to mankind.'

Children who grow up with attachment wounds and carry the residual effects of this trauma often don't recognise it as something that has shaped their lives. I would argue that interrupted primary attachment is probably one of the biggest traumas a person can carry – often because it's invisible and they have internalised the shame of not feeling loved so they believe the problem lies within them rather than being a reaction to something that happened to them.

All of this is without even factoring in our toxic modern environment – stress, lack of sleep, saturation in technology and a Western society that doesn't create space for periods and the menstrual cycle. It's far more common in Western societies for women to begin hating their bodies and cycles than not. Being female is a huge source of stress in and of itself, and no woman is immune to the soup we grow up swimming in. And then there's the system that's meant to heal us. Many of the women I see have experienced trauma at the hands of a well-meaning medical system. The first assault is the general lack of trauma-informed care, which fails to recognise traumatised people and ends up dismissing them or retraumatising them. If you have chronic pelvic pain or have been diagnosed with endometriosis, you may well have medical trauma from a prolonged lack of agency or power over your body and what has been done to you.

How did you get here?

Before you can look at healing your trauma and rewiring your nervous system to dial down pain, you have to look at how you got here. It's very important to emphasise that the aim of this is not to stay in the past or in the traumatising event but to gain insight and knowledge into how your body may have changed to keep you safe. From there you can begin to have compassion for yourself and learn your way back to a place of safety. Some people will do this by working with a therapist, while others can find their way back to safety with the help of a supportive community.

Before you do the following exercise, make sure you're in a safe place. Some of the prompts may trigger memories or bodily responses, especially if your traumas are unprocessed and your window of tolerance is narrow. This isn't about processing trauma, just beginning to recognise the things that may have shaped or changed your nervous system. Remember, you can utilise any of the tools in the previous chapter to bring you back into your window of tolerance if you notice yourself becoming dysregulated. You may wish to work through the exercise with your therapist if you have one.

Exercise: Journaling on your story

Start by thinking about whether there are things in your past or present that your body may have sensed as dangerous and pushed you into survival mode to cope with.

Although our nervous system is more likely to become stuck the earlier our exposure to stressful life events are (developmental trauma), sometimes our childhood and adolescence can be safe and supported and our life stressors come later. Many of my patients find writing about the challenges in their lives to be cathartic, as it helps to create a pathway to how their body may have adapted to

the place they are in now. Work through the journaling prompts
below, or use them to free-write on anything you feel is relevant
in your life up until this point. As you write, keep in mind the
question of safety throughout your life and whether your physical
and emotional needs were reliably being met.

Childhood
....
....

Adolescence
....
....

Adulthood
....
....

Recent times
....
....

Reflect on these questions
Did you feel safe to be yourself at home growing up?
....
....

What were and/or are your relationships like with your primary
caregivers?
....
....
....

Was there any illness, alcohol or drug abuse in your family growing up?

....

....

....

Did you or do you ever experience bullying or a feeling of being excluded at school?

....

....

....

Were there or are there high expectations for you to 'perform' or 'succeed' at school or work at the cost of other aspects of your physical or mental health?

....

....

....

Are you able to rest or do you feel the need to be constantly on the go and productive?

....

....

....

Do you feel able to be your authentic self without feeling rejected or persecuted, or do you regularly betray yourself for validation, love or acceptance?

....

....

....

What stories were you told about puberty and periods as a child? Were they generally positive or negative?

....

....

....

Did other female family members have a difficult relationship with their bodies or menstrual cycles?

....

....

....

Do you feel supported and able to care for yourself during your periods and take things slower if you need to, or do you feel the need to push through?

....

....

....

Have you had any invasive medical procedures or felt out of control or disempowered by encounters with the medical system?

....

....

....

Have you experienced physical, sexual or emotional abuse?

....

....

....

A powerful exercise

Writing your story can be helpful because it can pinpoint how your experiences have shaped you and your physical body through your nervous system's adaptations. Establishing a timeline of these adaptations allows you to match them to when your physical symptoms or pain began to develop. This can be very illuminating. It can often help you not only to understand why your body changed when it did, but also to cultivate compassion and gratitude for your body. It helped you survive when you needed it to. That's an incredible thing. Having this knowledge can help your body to remember that the past is over and it's safe to let go and return to a state where you can thrive once again.

Please note that even if your answers in this exercise indicate that you have lived through traumatic events, you may not necessarily be carrying that trauma in your body and living as a traumatised person. We each react differently to our circumstances, and many people are able to process stressful events and live optimally in the present, letting go of the effects of trauma on the body. This is what we're trying to achieve. Awareness is the first step on the path to recovery.

Working with a therapist can be invaluable

Some of you reading this book will already be working with a psychologist, psychotherapist or trauma specialist. Others may be only acknowledging potentially severe trauma for the first time. If you feel you need professional help to unpack difficult experiences, please reach out to a therapist experienced in trauma work. In his seminal work *The Body Keeps the Score*, Bessel van der Kolk writes that when it comes to helping traumatised people, it's important for the therapist to acknowledge and work with the body as well as thoughts and emotions. This is because the body and the brain cannot be separated, and what affects one affects the other.

A multidisciplinary approach

Renowned trauma expert, Bessel van der Kolk, recommends seeking out a therapist who specialises in some form of somatic therapy rather than just standard cognitive behavioural therapy (CBT), which has not been shown to be particularly effective for trauma when used alone. It's true that thoughts can change feelings that can affect the body, but ignoring the effects of trauma on the body means missing a huge part of the puzzle. Although there needs to be much more research on mind–body trauma therapy for chronic pain, if you recognise that trauma is a part of your story I would recommend a therapist who, along with CBT, works with some or all of the modalities below:

- somatic experiencing – the process of paying attention to the body: listening to the body without judgement or attaching fear of the future or memories of the past
- eye movement desensitisation and reprocessing (EMDR)
- neurofeedback
- relational therapy
- psychotherapy
- embodiment practices – including yoga and dance
- mindfulness and breath practices. (There is stacks of evidence that mindfulness improves pain and quality of life for people with chronic pain by rewiring pain pathways and helping people find their way back into a state of safety.)

Research consistently shows that for people with both chronic pain and trauma, a multidisciplinary approach is the best way forward. This is because it treats the changes in the brain and nervous system that lead to living in both a traumatised body and a body wired for pain. We know from Chapter 9 that the effects of trauma predispose people to developing chronic pain conditions as well as other health issues. The link is indisputable.

Leaving fear and pain behind

I believe that in order to heal chronic pain it's crucial to acknowledge, process and release the trauma you may have stored in your body. Obviously this isn't a one-time thing and it's gone for good. 'Doing the work' looks different for everyone, but when we understand that our body responds the way it does because what happened to us left an imprint, we can begin to carve new pathways so that we no longer respond from the fear and pain of the past. Healing is completely possible once we can connect the dots. If you're living with trauma, it's important to keep reminding yourself that it's not your fault and that your body is capable of healing if you have the support to return to a place of safety.

We've all had terrible or difficult things happen to us in varying degrees – in life we cannot expect to escape these things. But if we haven't allowed the stress to move through us or allowed our nervous system to return to safety, our nervous system will remain dysregulated. This keeps us stuck in the past, living on edge, unable to be fully alive in the present. Chronic nervous system dysregulation is often at the base of the pain iceberg (see page 170), affecting all our other bodily systems and leading to the *symptoms* we experience, including pelvic pain. Even if we reduce inflammation and immune system dysregulation by directly addressing the gut, working with anti-inflammatory supplements and so on, none of it will matter if we miss the big one. Over time, a chronically dysregulated nervous system will continue to sabotage any attempts to play whack-a-mole with symptoms.

Nervous system dysregulation and the development of neuroplastic pain are at the heart of most chronic pelvic pain. If we can address that, the body can usually find its way back to safety and homeostasis and heal itself. When pain is chronic, we sometimes need to dig down deep to find it. It's not just about *thinking* our way out of pain – top-down therapy – although that's part of retraining our brain. It's about *feeling* our way back to safety – through bottom-up therapy. This is about using our body to rewire our brain and pain pathways. It's not a quick or easy fix, but when you can achieve it, everything in life becomes easier. Not only will your pain be better, but so will your digestion, immune system, mood and relationships.

It's not about crushing pain or 'fighting the war' against endo, it's about coming back to the place in your body where you feel safe. This is not only where your gut, immune system and hormones function best, but also where joy, connection and vitality live.

I don't want you to 'fight' your pain – that just reinforces that there's something dangerous in your body and perpetuates a pain response. I want you to feel safe so you can listen to the story your body is trying to tell you. From there you can be and do the things that make your soul sing. When we try to push pain away, we start to catastrophise – spiralling into an anxious or depressed state in response to the fear of pain – which reinforces pathways in our brain that tell us we're in danger. But if we feel safe enough, we can start to get curious about pain and even befriend it (believe it or not) rather than fear it. This space is where the shift happens.

Understanding how our trauma and ongoing stress have changed our nervous system, brain and physical body means making sense of why we may be stuck. It also highlights our incredible power of neuroplasticity. If we start from a place of safety and stability, it's highly possible for us to find real healing and a way out of chronic pain.

Chapter summary

- Identifying the history of trauma and the stress your body is holding is an important part of understanding your pain story.
- Understanding how your pain system has become hypersensitive connects the dots, gives you answers and shows you a way out of pain.
- When you understand what you have been holding on to or trying to escape, you can finally begin the journey of letting it go.
- Working with a trauma therapist may be an important part of your healing.
- Feeling safe enough to go towards a pain sensation, rather than attempt to 'escape or fight', is key when it comes to reducing pain.

14

Rewiring pain pathways and reducing fear

By now I'm sure I've hammered home the idea that no part of us is separate from the other. Our brain and body work in unison through the bridge of our autonomic and somatic nervous systems (see Chapter 8). And we're not separate from our environment, which includes the nervous systems of the people around us. What happens in that environment changes our nervous system and hence our physiology. In order to address pelvic pain at its roots, we have to look beyond the pelvis and start in our nervous system. We have to befriend our nervous system and body, and instead of viewing our body or pain as the enemy, we need to start getting curious about it and questioning whether we have anything to fear now.

Fear drives chronic pain

A normal inflammatory process that in someone with a regulated nervous system and no fear may feel like mild discomfort because their danger-detection system is set to low, may feel excruciating to you because your danger detection is dialled up to 11/10. The analogy I often give my patients is that of a house alarm. A normally operating house alarm will go off and/or alert the police if someone throws a rock though the window or it detects someone breaking in. That's the alarm system doing its job to detect actual danger so that help arrives. In the body, we want our pain-pathway system to detect actual tissue damage – such as a burst appendix or a ruptured fallopian tube from an ectopic pregnancy – and alert our brain to the danger by producing a pain sensation because of active tissue damage.

But we don't want a house alarm system so sensitive that it goes off every five seconds when a leaf brushes against the window or the postie puts a letter in the mailbox. In this scenario the alarm system is faulty and is detecting danger everywhere where there is none. This is what happens in the body and brain of women with chronic pain. Even normal bodily sensations become perceived as painful, and potentially mildly painful ones such as a period can become unbearable.

As we saw in Chapter 7, this is known as pain system hyper-sensitivity and is always involved when pain persists. Because this is happening in the nervous system and the brain, then only addressing the pelvis – such as with surgery – will never be the complete answer. If you have chronic pelvic pain but you haven't addressed your nervous system and your pain alarm system, you'll still have pain, no matter what your diet is like, how many supplements you take or how many surgeries you have.

So how do we address this alarm system so that it becomes less jumpy? How do we rewire it to respond to actual danger signals rather than normal bodily sensations?

You're already well on the way

By simply getting to this point in the book, you've already begun to address the first few steps in rewiring your pain pathways.

Now that you know how chronic pain develops and that it's generally not due to ongoing tissue damage or danger, your fear regarding your pain may already be lower. You have also learnt that it's counterproductive to fear endometriosis – because endometriosis is not always associated with pain and many women have lesions with no issues. You know that ongoing pelvic pain usually involves:

- a dysregulated autonomic nervous system that turns up inflammation and leads to gut and immune system dysfunction
- upregulated pain pathways that amplify bodily sensations, including those of periods, which are a normal inflammatory process
- tense pelvic floor muscles
- fear and protective or avoidant behaviours.

None of these things are inherently scary, and when you understand them your fear starts to crumble. When you're given a map for navigating these causes you're empowered. Lots of research shows that chronic pain improves through pain education alone, because when the causes of pain remain mysterious, our subsequent feelings of helplessness leave us at the mercy of things happening inside our body that we don't understand – dialling up our fear and pain.

Modern pain science tells us that pain education is vital in improving the lives of people with chronic pain and should therefore be the start of any discussion of pain, including initial conversations about period pain. As fear always exacerbates pain, it's crucial to begin dialling it down from the very start. We also know that people who understand how their bodies work have lower pain levels than people with lower health literacy.

Understanding the role of the nervous system in the development and maintenance of chronic pain is the next part. You now understand why your nervous system changes to respond to your environment and how these changes, when they persist, upregulate pain pathways, alter gut and immune function, and drive inflammation and muscular dysfunction. You now know you're not broken or defective. You've just responded to an unsafe environment. By mapping out the path of your nervous system and the stressors you've encountered along the way, you can start to put the pieces together so that your pain begins to make total sense. You can now also see why approaching the problem from the tip of the iceberg down, rather than the ground up often fails, leaving more women feeling more hopeless than ever. And why doctors should be helping women return to equilibrium in their nervous system first.

The way things were meant to be

Prioritising a return to equilibrium in your nervous system hinges on the idea that in an ideal environment our body is supposed to function well without chronic and debilitating pain. Women were not born to need 15 supplements, multiple surgeries and a highly restrictive diet. When our nervous system feels safe, our body and mind are wired for health, repair, rest, connection and joy. Unfortunately, pharmaceutical and supplement companies rely on making us feel like health is elusive without them. While pharmaceuticals, supplements, herbs and sometimes surgery are tools in my toolbox, they are useless for chronic pain without first addressing the health and flexibility of the nervous system.

You might resonate with this. It's hard to remember to take all the supplements or make all the dietary changes asked of you on your chronic pain or endometriosis journey, especially when your nervous system is dysregulated. Most women could save a lot of money and make lasting change by working on calming their nervous system and pain pathways first. Many will find that when they're operating more often from their window of tolerance, their gut, immune system and pain pathways will be more regulated, meaning they don't need the other stuff. Beginning to understand the whole picture in this way makes you realise that *you* were never the problem. Your body has helped you survive under stress and you were never given the tools to find your way back out of survival mode. Your chronic pain is a danger signal gone awry.

Is your pain neuroplastic (brain-generated)?

I usually ask these questions to determine whether at least some of a patient's pain is neuroplastic:

- Is your pain the same all the time or is your pain worse when you're tired or under stress?
- Does your pain get worse when you're stuck in a high degree of fear about it?
- Have you had pain for greater than 3 months?

Most of my patients are able to notice that their pain tends to be worse when they're stressed, not sleeping, highly anxious, or fearful that their pain is the result of damage in their body. They can also recognise that when they're relaxed and feel safe in their life and their body, their pain tends to be better. They also notice that after we've talked about the origins of pain, their fear is lower and their pain is improved.

Rewiring your pain pathways

Now that you know that persistent pain is a sign of dysregulation, you can begin the path of healing that starts by using the tools in Chapter 12 to bring your body and your brain back from fight, flight or freeze into your window of tolerance. Rewiring your pain pathways and nervous system states is a simultaneous dance of bottom-up and top-down processing. This means we can't just think or feel our way out of pain – the most successful approach involves doing both at the same time. Our mind–body system is one entity and because of this, treatment needs to be similarly integrated. From now on, I want you to think about your pain through a lens of curiosity rather than fear.

You may already have seen a practitioner who understands the impact of fear on pain, and they may have recommended that you see a pain psychologist to help with rewiring these pathways and reducing underlying anxiety and fear. People tend to take the suggestion of a pain psychologist as implying the pain is all in their head and their doctor is being dismissive. But you now know that our thoughts are crucial in carving new neural pathways.

The downside, as you may already know, is that it can sometimes be nearly impossible to get an appointment with any psychologist, let alone one who specialises in pain. Given this issue, and the fact that as a gynaecologist I was seeing more and more women with chronic pain, I realised I had to upskill if I wanted to actually help them. I didn't feel it was enough to simply throw up my hands and say 'There's nothing I can do for you' or 'Go on this waiting list for six months to see a pain psychologist.' If I couldn't help these women, I would simply be the latest in a long line of practitioners who were unable to give them the answers or help they needed.

Pain reprocessing therapy

To help all my patients as quickly and effectively as possible, I learned pain reprocessing therapy, a method of rewiring the nervous system and brain that works on the concept of neuroplasticity to change the way the brain experiences pain. This new approach to neuroplastic chronic pain developed by Dr Howard Schubiner and Alan Gordon works by helping people understand that their pain is often not linked to tissue damage and by reducing their fear, which dials down protective responses and pain itself.

A 2022 clinical trial on patients with back pain, showed that with pain reprocessing therapy, 66 per cent of patients were pain-free or almost pain-free after the treatment compared with only 20 per cent for placebo treatment and 10 per cent for usual care. Most of the patients in the pain reprocessing therapy group maintained their results a year later.

Pain reprocessing therapy works on the idea that what we experience with chronic pain is in large part a reflection of what our brain predicts is going on inside our body based on past experiences and cultural conditioning rather than on actual internal sensations. In the words of neurologist Suzanne O'Sullivan, 'Predictive sensory processing can take expectations of pain and make pain.'

Our culture of fear of endometriosis as a chronic, incurable disease that always causes infertility, along with our culture of high stress and beliefs about periods being painful or a hassle, contributes to our sense of fear around pelvic pain. As we have seen, 80 per cent of endometriosis is superficial and may even be a normal part of the process of retrograde menstruation. We also know that a lot of women have endometriosis and no pain. And that a huge number of women with persistent pelvic pain, who may or may not have endometriosis, also have evidence of pain system hypersensitivity – upregulated pain pathways and brain-amplified pain.

This is exactly the kind of pain that's targeted by methods such as pain reprocessing therapy. It's also the kind of pain that can never be addressed with surgery. A recent New Zealand study showed that almost 75 per cent of women with pelvic pain had evidence of central sensitisation. These women were more likely to experience bowel and bladder pain, and were more likely to have been diagnosed with a mental health condition. If 75 per cent of women with pelvic pain have some element of neuroplastic pain, it's imperative that we start addressing the nervous system.

Once we accept that chronic pelvic pain is almost always due in part to changes in the brain and nervous system, we can use the science of neuroplasticity to unlearn and rewire these conditioned pain pathways.

If our body can learn pain, it can unlearn pain. That's the good news!

Using pain reprocessing therapy

After ruling out major structural issues like large ovarian cysts or deep endometriosis, or after conventional treatments for endometriosis have failed to bring relief from pain – chronic pain is almost always a sign of pain system hypersensitivity and not ongoing structural issues or tissue damage. When you have been diagnosed with pain system hypersensitivity there are three main components to using a technique such as pain reprocessing therapy to help retrain your pain pathways:

1. Safety re-appraisal – understanding that you're safe and there's nothing to fear.
2. Understanding that much of your pain is due to pain system hypersensitivity and is occurring with no or minimal tissue damage.
3. Learning somatic tracking – how to be in your body and turn towards the pain rather than away from it, and how to notice non-threatening sensations in your body.

Over time, this kind of practice helps to remind your body that you're safe and teaches your brain to dial down the perception of danger so that it doesn't need to produce a pain sensation.

Once you've seen a doctor and they've ruled out anything sinister and confirmed that some of your pain is due to these learned neural pathways, you can try pain reprocessing therapy at home.

Exercise: Pain reprocessing therapy
Don't try this if you have really severe pain or you're in a bad place emotionally and are unable to come into a relaxed state using the techniques in Chapter 12. It's best to do this exercise for the first time when your pain is at a manageable level – less than a 5/10.

Find a safe and relaxed place and a comfortable position.

Step 1: Remember you are safe
Remind yourself that despite the pain there's nothing dangerous happening in your body.

Remind yourself of all the physiological reasons periods can be uncomfortable – the uterine muscles contracting, prostaglandins and inflammation, the pelvic floor and sensitised pain pathways.

Remind yourself that **none** of these things is dangerous.

Remind yourself that you've seen a doctor, you've had an ultrasound scan and there's no permanent damage occurring.

Remind yourself that if you've had endometriosis diagnosed and removed, it doesn't need to cause pain and can be managed by supporting your immune system, reducing inflammation and coming to a safe place in your nervous system.

Remind yourself that if you've had a normal ultrasound scan, any endometriosis you do have is likely to be superficial, and that many women with no pain symptoms have the same findings.

Remind yourself that some mild superficial endometriosis may be akin to normal wear and tear of a menstruating body and is nothing to fear.

A mantra that many of my patients find helpful is 'I'm sore, but I'm safe.'

Step 2: Lean in to the pain sensation

Come to a relaxed place in your body. Close your eyes. Start by using a deep breathing technique such as two inhales through the nose and a long exhale through the mouth. Now turn towards your pain with curiosity. Simply observe the sensation without fear and without attaching meaning to it. Now you know that you are safe, it's okay to pay gentle attention to the pain. Observe it inside your body just as though you were at the ballet. Observe the sensation as if you're observing a dancer on the stage.

Notice the intensity of the sensation.

Notice the quality of the sensation – is it a tightness, a heaviness, a dull ache, a sharp pain?

See what else you can notice. Does the sensation have a colour? Does the sensation move, come and go, or is it static?

Get curious and notice it. Befriend it. Remember there's nothing to fear. It's simply your brain misinterpreting a sensation in your body as dangerous and making a pain sensation to protect you.

Keep breathing as you continue to notice it – two inhalations through the nose and one long exhale through the mouth.

Step 3: Leaning in to other sensations

Now gently turn your attention towards a positive or neutral sensation in your body. It might be the feeling of your breath, it could be a sound around you, it could be the feeling of your head gently resting on a pillow, the comforting feeling of a heat pack on your pelvis, a pleasant smell like an essential oil diffuser. If you can't find a neutral or positive sensation, make one by rubbing your palms together, stroking your belly, touching your tongue to the roof of your mouth, humming, or feeling your clothing resting on your body. Stay with one of these sensations and feel it deeply for about 10 seconds.

Often when I'm guiding a patient through this practice, we go back to the pain sensation at the end and find that it has moved, changed, lessened or gone altogether. This is further proof that the pain is not due solely or at all to a structural issue or ongoing tissue damage but is neuroplastic.

CASE STUDY: LOUISE

Louise was in her late twenties when she came to see me after having had daily pelvic pain for the past six months. She had been a lawyer but had moved into a less stressful and more satisfying job a few years earlier after experiencing significant burnout in her legal career.

In the past, Louise had been diagnosed with premenstrual dysphoric disorder, an extreme form of premenstrual syndrome that can cause severe sadness, hopelessness and irritability or anger. The majority of her symptoms had abated, however, after she changed jobs and reduced her stress levels. Although Louise had experienced sexual and physical violence in her childhood and adolescence that led to complex PTSD, she was now in a healthy, loving long-term relationship and had a lot

---

of understanding about how trauma had affected her, having spent a long time with a trauma therapist. She had really good insight into this, had done a lot of healing and was in a really good place.

Her pain was slightly worse with her periods, but she described it as occurring on most days. She was worried about endometriosis. She didn't experience pain with sex or bowel motions or in her bladder, and she had a normal high-resolution ultrasound. When we talked about the timeline of her pain and its relation to other events in her life, she realised that it started when her partner went away for work. He'd just begun a job working in the mines and was away for weeks at a time. She realised, when we talked about hypervigilance in response to previous trauma, that although she had done a lot of healing, she relied on her partner for co-regulation and that her sense of danger perhaps went up when he left for work.

We did a session of pain reprocessing therapy in a very relaxed place on a yoga mat under our centuries-old fig tree at Vera. She started the session with 5/10 pain and ended it with no pain at all. Because Louise already understood how trauma can affect the nervous system, and had come to me with normal imaging, she responded really well when we could re-establish the sense of safety and stability in her body that she was missing while her partner was away.

This kind of practice is known as top-down processing – using awareness, thinking and psycho-education to change our brain and then our experience of pain in the body. Just as with trauma, the best therapy for chronic pain also includes bottom-up processing – using the body to communicate a sense of safety to the brain.

Movement as therapy

Since at least 80 per cent of the messages travelling along our vagus nerve go from the body to the brain, what happens in the body can change the way our brain works, not just the other way around. This is why things like yoga improve chronic pain and can help people who live in a traumatised, dysregulated body. Bessel van der Kolk showed in his research that yoga can positively affect the brain and help people learn how to feel safe in their body. He showed that heart-rate variability increased in many people doing yoga, indicating decreased stress and improved resilience. Yoga for patients with chronic pelvic pain has shown to improve pain and increase in quality of life compared to patients undertaking conventional treatment only.

Yoga practice has been shown to increase levels of brain-derived neurochemicals that are associated with reduced pain states. Other forms of movement can do the same thing, which is why movement is so important. Studies have also shown improvements in chronic pain with all forms of dance therapy. Other forms of movement, such as music, drumming, qigong and martial arts also have a big role to play.

Many of these things are ancient and have been practised as part of a healthy lifestyle that connects people to their bodies, their community and their sense of something greater than themselves. There's a reason why healing in many cultures around the world involves movement, dance and music – because they connect us back to our bodies and allow the completion of the stress cycle so that we can release trauma from the body. In our Western societies we've lost this critical step in mobilising trauma to allow its release from the body.

Exercise: Dance

Notice how you feel in your body.

Put your favourite high-energy music on and dance like no one's watching for just one song.

Now notice how your body feels. How does your mood feel? Do you feel the release of stress hormones? Does your body feel different from before you moved? How? Do you feel less pain?

Leaving a freeze state through movement

Being stuck in a freeze state disconnects us from our body, prevents healing from trauma and perpetuates pain. We need to engage the body through movement back into safety. Writing about somatic experiencing, psychologist Peter Levine explains that for many people, movement completes the stress response by moving them from shutdown and allowing their body to settle back into a healthy regulated parasympathetic or ventral vagal state. Without this, they stay stuck in collapse or freeze.

Moving the body, allowing for deep belly breathing and paying attention to the breath all activate the vagus nerve, which sends messages of safety to the brain. If you really were in danger you would take shallow breaths – which is what many of us do – reinforcing a mistaken sense of danger to the brain and perpetuating fear and chronic pain. So taking deep breaths sends a message of safety through our vagus nerve to our brain, dialling down the fear–pain response.

Pelvic floor therapy: the vital next step

Deep breaths through the relaxation of the diaphragm are intrinsically connected with movement of the pelvic floor. The thoracic diaphragm in the chest – the muscle that contracts and expands to allow for inhalation and exhalation – sits under the lungs. Think of it as the top of a can. The sides of the can are the sides of our body, our back and our belly, the bottom is the pelvic floor. When the diaphragm relaxes, so too does the pelvic floor. When the diaphragm is constantly contracted and unrelaxed through rapid shallow breathing, so too is the pelvic floor, which leads to pelvic floor muscle tension and pelvic pain.

When discussing bottom-up therapy in my practice, I talk about the benefits of yoga, dance, movement, breath and embodied somatic therapy. But the foundation of this kind of therapy for women with chronic pelvic pain is pelvic floor therapy with a pelvic floor physiotherapist acting as a guide to bring awareness back into the body. Many women with persistent pelvic pain find this confronting, particularly if they've experienced trauma and don't believe their body is a safe space to inhabit.

But through awareness, an experienced pelvic floor physiotherapist can help you safely navigate back to your body, so that you can meet yourself again and begin the process of embodiment. To be embodied is to be connected to your body and aware of how your emotions affect it, including the state of your nervous and muscular system. When you become aware of how your body feels at any given moment, you can begin to notice dysfunctional patterns that may be contributing to your brain's perception of danger. By learning a different way of being that fosters a sense of safety in the body, you are changing your brain from the bottom up.

Chapter summary

- Pain education and a solid understanding about how pain system hypersensitivity or neuroplastic pain works is vital in reducing fear associated with pain.
- Pain reprocessing therapy is one tool I use to retrain the nervous system to dial down pain, but many pain psychologists use similar tools including somatic tracking – paying attention without fear or judgement to bodily sensations.
- Pain reprocessing therapy uses pain education, relaxation and somatic tracking (paying attention to sensations in the body) to dial down pain.
- Reframing the way we think about pain and becoming curious rather than fearful is key.
- Trying to escape from pain perpetuates more pain.

15

Connecting the brain and body with pelvic floor therapy

Almost all the women I see with chronic pelvic pain, and many with period pain, have pelvic floor tension. This simply means that the muscles lining the floor of the pelvis – through which our vagina, rectum and urethra pass – have become overly tight. Tight muscles become sore muscles and a source of tension in the body. Many women are surprised when I mention the pelvic floor as a contributing player in their pelvic pain. Most women have only ever thought of the pelvic floor as something that becomes weak after childbirth and can result in bladder leakage when we cough or sneeze. They're often shocked to learn that these same muscles can also cause problems when they become too tense and lose the ability to relax, as is frequently the case with pelvic pain.

How pelvic floor tightness begins

Most of you will have experienced what tight muscles in other parts of your body feel like – neck, shoulders, back and jaw are good examples. You're also likely to understand how muscle tension can spread and be felt in nearby areas of the body, as is often the case with tension headaches caused by neck and shoulder tension. You might have experienced or understand the concept of muscular spasm. Back spasms can be intensely painful. Muscular spasm is likely to occur the tighter or more contracted a muscle is.

Just as these muscles can become tight or go into painful spasm, so too can the muscles of the pelvic floor, which will be experienced as chronic pelvic pain, intense period pain, painful sex, constipation, painful or incomplete bladder emptying or sharp stabbing pains with spasms. I joke with my patients that no one has ever come to see me complaining of 'pelvic floor muscle tightness and pain' the way you might go to your doctor or physiotherapist with a tight neck and shoulders. They come with pelvic pain instead.

Although pelvic floor tightness is often referred to under the umbrella of pelvic floor dysfunction, I often bristle at that description, because most of the time your pelvic floor has become overactive for a good reason, not because you are inherently dysfunctional. The process of those muscles becoming tight frequently starts as a subconscious effort to protect you. It might begin in response to painful periods – when the body registers a stimulus that it deems dangerous – and then become a conscious immobilisation of the muscles because it seems dangerous to move or it will hurt more if you move. The sorer and tighter the muscles become, the more ingrained those protective behaviours can also become.

Most women with pelvic pain will be able to describe how they 'double over' at times and become 'crippled with pain', often retreating to bed where they avoid movement and remain curled up in a ball. These behaviours, while totally understandable, not only result in further muscle tightness but also reinforce the pain pathways that drive chronic pain by cementing the belief that there really is danger. This creates a muscular–neural bidirectional feedback loop where your brain gets the message from the protective behaviours that there is danger and so it should produce a pain signal to help protect you, while immobilisation increases muscular contraction and the likelihood of muscle spasm, both of which drive pain.

The muscles can also become tense when we're under chronic stress – just as we're more likely to get muscular tension in the neck, shoulders or jaw when we're stressed. Women especially store a lot of old trauma in the pelvis.

CASE STUDY: MARGARET

Margaret was 23 when she came to see me after two years of increasing period pain, ovulation pain, pain with sex and generalised pelvic pain on most days. She reported having fairly pain-free periods until the past few years. She had some symptoms of IBS but no pain using her bowels or her bladder.

Margaret reported no history of trauma, just social anxiety and a tendency to worry. She told me her bruxism – jaw clenching – was so severe she had broken teeth and required a night guard and Botox in her jaw to relieve her mouth pain. Margaret now worked in retail, but just before her pain started she had been studying for a physiotherapy degree, an experience she found too stressful and that led to a period of burnout. She felt mostly quite relaxed now and was in a loving stable relationship. In her history, Margaret mentioned that she'd had a melanoma removed just before her pain started but she didn't tell me where.

She had a normal pelvic ultrasound with no evidence of deep endometriosis. On examination, the first thing that struck me was a large scar over her labia majora – the outer lips of the labia. Margaret told me this was where the melanoma had been removed and that a complication with an infection meant the wound broke apart and her doctor had to resuture it. As she recounted this, she told me how traumatic it was at the time – not only the pain and being sutured 'down there' while she was awake, but also her worry about cancer.

When I examined her pelvic floor, I found it to be holding a lot of tension, with lots of pain and trigger points when I gently palpated the muscles. Her pain was all in the pelvic floor, with no pain around her uterus or ovaries.

Even though Margaret had studied physiotherapy for two years, she hadn't learnt that pelvic floor muscle tension can lead to pelvic pain. While she knew that the tension she held in her jaw led to headaches and neck pain, she had no awareness when it came to her pelvic floor. She was surprised to learn that there's often a correlation between tension in the jaw and in the pelvic floor – when one is tight the other is also likely to be holding tension because of shared fascial connections. She had also never connected the dots between the trauma she experienced over the melanoma in her vulva and the onset of her pain.

Other factors involved in pelvic floor tension

Some women who do a lot of high-intensity exercise, Pilates, gymnastics, ballet or horse riding can also develop pelvic floor tension due to increased activation of their pelvic floor and adductor muscles. While these activities can be really enjoyable for many women, if the pelvic floor becomes too tense without being able to relax, pain can be more likely. Having a strong core is important for optimal functioning, however learning to relax it is just as important.

The other and all too frequent reason for an overactive pelvic floor is sexual assault or abuse. In this scenario, the pelvic floor is literally acting appropriately to protect you. For me it almost sounds offensive to use the phrase pelvic floor dysfunction in this situation. It's not dysfunctional. It's a survival response and there's nothing wrong with your body if it reacted to protect you in this way. What is very wrong is what happened to you and what happens to far too many women. But there's nothing wrong with you if this is your situation. I need you to know that your body is amazing and it did what it needed to do to protect you when there was danger, when you weren't safe. Your brain didn't get it wrong. The danger was out there. It wasn't your body. You were violated, and your body is a strong and incredible warrior that armoured up to get you through it.

If you've experienced sexual trauma and as a result have extreme difficulty having sex at all due to pelvic floor muscle tightness, you may have been diagnosed with vaginismus. This word simply means tight pelvic floor muscles, but as a diagnosis it leaves women feeling defective rather than telling it like it is – an appropriate survival response to sexual trauma. Obviously, when the pelvic floor muscles are too tense, it can make penetrative sex difficult or impossible, while also contributing to painful periods and chronic pelvic pain. The pelvic floor muscles are carrying all that tension and trauma because they're on guard, so to speak, and ready for danger. It's a defensive mechanism that, over time, can cause problems.

I often see a similar issue when women have experienced medical trauma – painful pelvic exams, not feeling safe, or having no power or control over what was being 'done to them'. Too often to count, the pelvic floor is tense because of all these factors.

The multidisciplinary approach works

Unfortunately, as in so many areas of women's health, we need more research into physiotherapy for pelvic pain. A few studies have shown some benefit, mostly in women who are undergoing the physiotherapy treatment as part of a multidisciplinary approach to their pain.

As for many therapies that aren't as cut and dried as a pill versus a placebo, especially hands-on therapies and those that rely on a good patient–therapist relationship, there are lots of barriers to designing good-quality studies. These things are much harder to measure in terms of quantitative data, not to mention the cost of such trials to run when there's no pharmaceutical company to fund them. Having said that, a recent 2022 systematic review showed that three out of four randomised control trials of physiotherapy for pelvic floor overactivity showed significant improvements in terms of pain.

I'm so convinced that tight pelvic floor muscles are linked to pain, and that a good trauma-informed and holistic physiotherapist can make a huge difference to a woman's healing, that I've designed my clinical space around a multidisciplinary team that includes a physiotherapist. I believe so strongly in the value of this approach to women with pain that I left my previous clinic when allied health services such as physiotherapy, psychology and nutrition were cut.

Are you holding tension in your pelvic floor?

If you have chronic pelvic pain, very painful periods, intense stabbing pains, and pain or difficulty with sex, inserting a tampon or menstrual cup, bowel movements or bladder emptying, it's highly likely that you have some element of pelvic floor muscle overactivity.

By now you probably know that I'm not big on labelling every symptom a woman might have as a disease when it's usually a sign of a greater issue – namely an upregulated nervous system. For this reason, I don't think of pelvic floor overactivity as a diagnosis in itself – it represents the way your body has responded to your external or internal environment to keep you safe. Understanding how your body has got here gives you greater compassion for yourself and a roadmap back to a place of regulation where safety resides. For this reason, identifying pelvic floor tension is really important in understanding pain and as part of holistic healing.

You don't *need* a pelvic floor examination: it's your choice

Many women are put off going to see a pelvic floor physiotherapist because they're worried about a pelvic examination, which is completely understandable when you think about how they may have felt unsafe or triggered in the past.

It's important to know that a pelvic floor exam is not necessary at all, and that there's plenty you can do to bring awareness to your pelvic floor and learn how to feel safe and relaxed without any internal examinations.

I do offer to do a pelvic exam when I think there's a significant component of overactivity, because very often no one has looked at this piece of the puzzle and it can be very helpful for a woman to learn where her tension is being held and how that contributes to her pelvic pain. I do this, however, with the following caveats:

- never with young girls who have not been sexually active or not used a tampon.
- only after obtaining informed consent – explaining why an exam might be helpful as information gathering in order to determine what's contributing to pain. To do this, I explain the purpose of the exam and ask 'Is this okay?' while also explaining that it's also okay to say no altogether. If it's the first appointment, I add that we can leave it until another day, if at all.
- if I'm already aware of previous trauma that could cause an exam to be triggering, only after we've worked together to ensure that she has established a sense of safety and stability.
- only after creating a safe and nurturing environment by offering a support person if she needs, and by using things such as music, low lighting and essential oils to help her ground herself in her body and remain safely present.
- only after ensuring that she knows she's in charge and feels safe enough to be able to say stop at any time and I will listen.

It's of paramount importance in the healing of pelvic pain that you feel safe and in control first and foremost, and this approach should be what we expect as women.

If you don't feel comfortable with a pelvic exam, there are lots of other ways a physiotherapist can assess your pelvic floor, including:

- observing breathing patterns. As the pelvic floor and diaphragm are intimately connected, many women with pelvic floor over-activity have tightness and dysfunctional movement patterns in their abdominal wall as well. Many will tend to breathe up into their chest rather than allowing their diaphragm to fully relax for full diaphragmatic or belly breathing.
- observing your vulva and perineum with a mirror and watching for muscle contraction or the muscles around the anus and vagina drawing in – almost like a turtle drawing its head into its shell in retreat. The mirror helps you connect with what's happening in your own body rather than just being examined by someone outside of you. It brings awareness to your pelvic floor when you might usually have no conscious awareness that you are contracting your muscles. This is a type of biofeed-back – a technical sounding word that just means embodiment. Biofeedback is the process of being in your body and noticing what you're feeling.
- using ultrasound, which can be transabdominal (over your tummy) or transperineal (over the perineum – the area between the anus and vagina). Ultrasound can provide another avenue for biofeedback because it allows the physiotherapist to identify the muscle on the screen and for you watch it change as you contract and relax your muscles. This helps ensure that you're actually relaxing the correct muscles. Once you've experienced the difference between contracted muscles and relaxed ones, you'll have the skills to actively relax when you sense your pelvic floor is tightening in the future.
- over time and only if you're comfortable, manual pelvic floor therapy with a physiotherapist. Some women find this helpful, but it's not absolutely necessary.

Pelvic floor physiotherapy
Good pelvic floor therapy is not just kneading out tight spots in the muscle (trigger points) as it might be for back or shoulder

pain, for example. It aims to learn not just about the muscles but to understand the story behind your pelvic floor overactivity. It's about you understanding and becoming aware of the messages between your brain and nervous system and your pelvic floor, and deepening the relationship between you and your body. It's about guiding you safely back into your body to start to rewire those neural pathways that are keeping you stuck in chronic pain.

All too often when a woman begins working with a good pelvic floor physiotherapist, it's the first time she has paid attention with curiosity rather than fear to what's going on in her pelvic floor. I believe so strongly that you cannot heal pelvic pain until you feel safe enough to be in your body that my multidisciplinary holistic clinic includes heart-centred, trauma-informed pelvic physiotherapists who play a key role in helping women understand the link between trauma, their brain, their pelvic floor and their experience of pelvic pain.

To help you understand the importance of pelvic floor therapy for pelvic pain I asked our incredible pelvic floor physiotherapist at Vera Women's Wellness, Brooke, to share some of her practical wisdom. While it's ideal to have an expert guide to help you navigate this part of your journey, there are practices you can begin right now today to help you deepen your connection to and relationship with your pelvic floor and thus yourself.

Healing through connection to self
by Brooke Dobó, pelvic floor physiotherapist

Pelvic floor muscle connection
The first step to pelvic floor muscle rehabilitation is your own connection to this part of your body.

Physiotherapists are trained in biofeedback, the clinical term for embodiment. This refers to strategies that enable connection of your brain to an area of your body by utilising your senses. The female pelvic floor can be a challenging area for the brain to perceive, as unlike a biceps muscle, for example, the movement cannot be witnessed on the outside.

Experienced women's health physiotherapists have come up with creative ways to improve awareness of the pelvic floor, which ultimately improves motor control. This gives you the ability not only feel to your muscles contract on demand, but also to relax them following a contraction. Furthermore, improving your ability to sense how your pelvic floor feels enables you to acknowledge when tension may be rising there (for example, during a long, stressful day on your feet) and gives you the power to consciously let that tension go when needed. This may seem like a foreign concept, but it's achievable with determination and practice, and guidance from a trained professional.

It's very difficult to heal an area of your body that your mind isn't connected to, hence the importance of this first step. You may not find it easy for several different reasons. Here are some examples of pelvic floor muscle biofeedback:

- visual: looking at your vulva in a mirror and watching for movement of the perineum as you contract your pelvic floor muscle – this is often the best place to start your connection to this area of your body (see the guided activity on the following page).
- visual: working with a pelvic health physiotherapist to visualise pelvic floor muscle movement using a real-time ultrasound on your lower abdomen (or sometimes perineum) – you can observe the base of the bladder move up and down with muscle contraction and relaxation.
- visual/audible: using one of various Bluetooth insertable devices connected to a smart phone app to visualise and 'hear' pelvic floor muscle activity.
- visual/audible: using an electromyography (EMG) biofeedback machine with a trained physiotherapist. The EMG measures electrical activity within the muscles using either electrodes placed on the perineum or an inserted vaginal or anal probe.

- tactile: feeling the movement of your perineum with your hand on it while attempting to contract your pelvic floor muscle. If you're comfortable, you can also insert a clean, lubricated finger into your vagina to feel pelvic floor muscle activation.
- tactile/visual: using one of various insertable devices that enable you to feel the squeeze within the vagina as you contract your pelvic floor. Some have indicators that point out correct contraction and relaxation.

There are many reasons why women are not aware of their pelvic space. Firstly, a lack of education has led to women, particularly older generations, not knowing what their anatomy looks like – they've never taken a look at their clitoris, urethral or vaginal openings or anus. This means the brain has insufficient information about the muscles and therefore muscle control around this area, which can often cause issues relating to the bowel, bladder and sexual function. Moreover, we live in a society that has fostered shame among women regarding their genitals, further disconnecting them from their bodies.

Here are a few practical exercises that may help you begin the journey of pelvic floor (re)connection, awareness and relaxation.

Exercise: Guided mirror observations

Be curious. Grab a mirror. This may be a small handheld mirror, a freestanding mirror, or perhaps a full-length mirror. If you can source a mirror with a small light, this is ideal for improved visual acuity. Otherwise you might like to use a lamp or torch. Find a comfortable position where you can visualise your vulva in your mirror of choice – it may take a few minutes to find the perfect spot depending on what's available to you. Some suggestions are: lying reclined on a bed with pillows behind your back and supporting your knees either side, or sitting, with knees bent, on a towel on the floor of your bedroom in front of a full-length mirror with the support of the bed or a couch behind you.

Firstly, simply observe. Then notice any thoughts, feelings or emotions that arise. Without judgement, acknowledge those thoughts and, if necessary, ask yourself why you think or feel this way. If this is your first time and you're feeling uncomfortable, you may like to stop there for your first attempt. If you are feeling okay, you may like to take a closer look by separating the outer labia with clean fingers – these are the outer folds of tissue that may or may not have pubic hair on them. If this is your first time, or if it's been a while, take time to examine your vulva and identify your anatomy: outer and inner labia, clitoris, urethral opening, vaginal opening, perineum and anus. You might find using a diagram helpful.

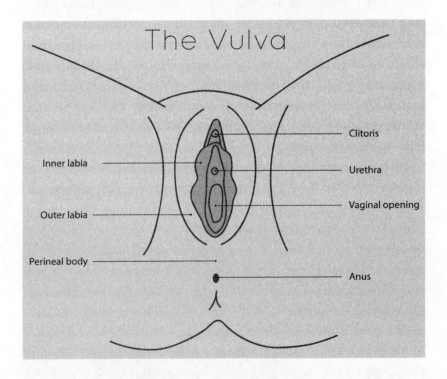

The Vulva

Clitoris

Inner labia

Urethra

Vaginal opening

Outer labia

Perineal body

Anus

Notice the different colours, shapes and sizes of the tissues. Take note of the amount of lubrication and vaginal discharge.

Then, tighten your pelvic floor muscles (think about holding on to wind or urine) and observe if there's any movement of the perineum. This is the tissue between your vaginal opening and anus and is where the pelvic floor muscles meet. With a correct contraction, you will see the perineum squeeze up inside the body, with perhaps a nodding down of the clitoris and a squeeze/'wink' of the anus. Everything then returns to its resting position as you relax. This movement may be subtle or obvious. You may see no movement at all, or perhaps the perineum moves down instead of rising up.

If you're not sure if you're contracting (or relaxing) correctly, don't become frustrated. This is very common, and the important thing is that you've taken the first step in enabling (training) your brain to correctly control these muscles. If you've been disconnected from these muscles for a long time, it can take a while to make the reconnection.

A pelvic health physiotherapist will be able to facilitate this connection. If you plan on seeing a pelvic health physiotherapist, this is a great activity to perform before your appointment, so you have an improved understanding of your level of confidence in pelvic floor muscle control.

Exercise: Diaphragmatic breathing

An experienced pelvic health physiotherapist will suggest that learning how to breathe correctly is the key to full-body engagement and ultimate connection to your pelvic floor muscles. With practice, this is an extremely helpful tool in pelvic floor muscle relaxation, and is often one of the first exercises a pelvic health physiotherapist will give you.

If you have an opportunity to watch a baby or toddler sleep, observe the way they breathe. You'll notice that they use their diaphragm muscle below the lungs, visible as a gentle rise and fall of their abdomen. This is the way we're designed to breathe when in a resting state. We tend to lose this pattern as we grow and transform into adults, distracted by constant daily life stressors. Being caught up in an ever-engaged sympathetic (fight or flight) nervous system means that we use our chest accessory muscles to breathe and our diaphragm becomes locked up, along with our abdominal and pelvic floor muscles.

You can perform diaphragmatic breathing exercises in any position at any time of the day. If this is a new concept to you or you're after some guidance on how to breathe correctly, here's a great place to start:

1. Lie comfortably on your back, fully supported by a bed, couch or yoga mat. Use pillows for support under your head and knees, to enable complete relaxation.
2. Place one hand on your chest and one hand on your lower belly.
3. Take a few slow deep inhales – notice where the air seems to travel – which hand is moving the most?
4. After a few breaths, aim to not move your top hand, but rather your belly – this does not mean pushing the abdomen out – it's a release and expansion of your abdominal muscles (which are linked in with the pelvic floor muscles as part of the core network).
5. Continue to breathe deeply into your pelvis, visualising an opening up of your pelvic muscles on each inhalation and complete softening on each exhalation.

It's important to practise diaphragmatic breathing regularly or preferably daily. Not only will this help reduce tension within your pelvic floor and abdominal muscles, but it will also:

- instil a feeling of calm during a busy day. This is why it's important to practise this exercise when you're feeling relaxed – so that it's easier to perform when you need it in stressful situations.
- down-regulate and calm the nervous system. This is one of the first exercises taught during cognitive behavioural therapy (CBT) for dealing with daily life stressors.
- activate your vagus nerve – in other words engage your parasympathetic nervous system (rest and digest) state

- *gently massage the colon, stimulating the gentle movement of food through your digestive tract.*

Three to five relaxed, slow belly breaths before getting out of bed is a beautiful way to start each day. Starting your day in a calm state sets you up for success, no matter how chaotic things may be with family, work, social engagements, commitments and so on. It also helps activate your rest and digest state, moving energy to your digestive system, which can help with opening your bowels first thing in the morning.

Body scan exercise
This is a useful exercise to help you to come into your body and notice any areas that may be holding tension. You can do it at any time of the day, in any position, in any location. It can also help you tune in to any protective postures you may be holding and improve your awareness of the way you move.

1. *Close your eyes or soften your gaze and begin with a few slow, deep breaths.*
2. *Bring your awareness to the top of your head.*
3. *Slowly shift your attention all the way down your body, taking time to focus on each area: scalp, facial muscles, ears, mouth, tongue, jaw, neck, chest, shoulders, arms, wrists, hands, fingers, back, abdomen, pelvis, hips, thighs, knees, lower legs, ankles, feet, toes.*
4. *You may like to breathe into each area and notice any sensations that arise. Aim to relax each part of your body as you scan along.*
5. *Once you've reached your toes, repeat the exercise, this time a little faster, to ensure each area has remained relaxed.*

Minimising protective behaviours
When we have pain, we're more likely to self-protect or subconsciously tighten our muscles or avoid certain movements out of fear of pain. These behaviours can lead to more muscle contraction

and more pain, and reinforce the concept of 'danger' to the brain. Pelvic floor therapy can help minimise the pattern of these behaviours through:

- connection exercises to become aware of these behaviours
- quick body scan exercises throughout the day
- 'Stop, Drop and Flop' reminders – practise throughout the day as a reminder to actively let go of the pelvic floor. How to:
  1. Stop – sit or lie in a relaxed position.
  2. Drop – pull the pelvic floor up like stopping a flow of urine and then gently release.
  3. Flop – release your abdominals and let them go floppy and relaxed.
  4. Spend a few minutes enjoying deep belly breathing.
- learning to breathe correctly, which will break down habitual muscle-tensing patterns such as holding in the abdominal and/ or pelvic floor muscles all day
- following #stopsuckingitin on Instagram to shift the mindset that we need flat tummies.

What pelvic floor physiotherapy should be

If you have a good pelvic floor physiotherapy session with an experienced heart-centred, trauma-informed therapist, you should:

- walk out of the clinic feeling heard and relieved that your goals are achievable, and empowered with a plan for how to begin the journey towards reaching them
- leave with practical information on how to connect to your body and begin moving it in a way that feels good.

You shouldn't:

- walk out of the clinic feeling uncertain, scared or defeated
- be given an exercise program prescription that's unattainable or unenjoyable.

I've seen remarkable results with holistic, trauma-informed pelvic floor physiotherapy that aims to go beyond tight muscles to helping women understand why they are storing tension, unravel old trauma and patterns of protection, and seek to establish a positive connection to their body. It's really about starting on the path to becoming an embodied woman. Not only have I seen countless women improve or resolve pelvic pain, but I've also seen them transform into women who live safely in their bodies and can even come to a place of enjoyment and pleasure within their bodies. This is what we should be aiming for: not just the absence of pain, but the ability to be safely present in the body – that place in our nervous system where we can experience connection and joy.

CASE STUDY: EVA

Eva was 20 when she came to see me with severe period pain and sharp stabbing pain that left her bedbound at times. The Pill did not really help the pain and she was suffering with troubling side effects such as spotting, low mood and libido, and painful sex. She felt a burning pain or stinging with sex and had been on the Pill since almost her first period due to painful, irregular periods.

Eva's high-quality pelvic ultrasound was normal. When she gave me permission to examine her vulva, I found the skin to be quite thin, likely due to the hormonal effects of long-term Pill use. She decided to come off the Pill and try a Mirena IUD instead (which was inserted under general anaesthetic so as not to further traumatise her or her pelvic floor). This would still give her contraception and lighter or non-existent periods, but would allow her brain and ovaries to talk to each other so that she could make her own testosterone, progesterone and oestrogen again, in the hope of improving her mood, libido and painful vulva.

Because of the pain she was experiencing with sex, her pelvic floor muscles had become overactive and tight as a reasonable protective bodily response. In addition to switching from the Pill to the Mirena IUD, I recommended some topical oestrogen and local anaesthetic cream for the skin on her vulva to help with re-oestrogenisation. I also suggested some visits with our pelvic floor physiotherapist, Brooke, whose wisdom you have just read.

When I saw Eva several months later she had far less period pain and stabbing pain, and no further pain with sex. Whereas before she had been terrified to get a period because she was afraid of the pain – which would trigger pelvic floor spasm, unconscious protective behaviours and a pain spiral – now she was getting a light monthly period with her Mirena and actually found she looked forward to it.

It's not like she had no pain at all. She still noticed some cramping around her period, especially if she was really stressed or hadn't been moving very much. The changes in the way she described her experience with her pain were really profound. During her pelvic floor physiotherapy sessions with Brooke and her consultations with me, Eva had learnt about all the amazing things happening inside her pelvis. She now knew that she didn't need to be afraid, that she could be curious instead. This led to changes in the language she used to describe her sensations, and almost a feeling of awe and curiosity rather than fear when she leaned in to her pain.

She learned to notice what was happening in her pelvic floor when she felt a sensation such as pain or experienced intense stressful emotions. Through that awareness, she learned she could connect to her body and use strategies such as breath, stretches, visualisation or reminding herself that she was safe. By doing this, she didn't eliminate all pain, but the meaning she gave to her pain changed. She was able to use the sensation of pain to realise when she was out of alignment or in a survival nervous system state. She could then use the tools Brooke taught her to deepen the connection to her body and navigate her way back to her safe ventral vagal state – where it was okay to relax her pelvic floor, reduce the signals of danger sent to her brain and, as a result, change her experience of pain.

When she saw me a little later, she told me that her last period had been a bit heavier and a little more painful, but this hadn't bothered her because she had the tools to manage it. She was actually happy to see me despite this recent period, because she thought she may have had a sensation of ovulating, and through all her recent education was excited about the prospect of her ovaries beginning to work again. She had been able to tune in to her emotions, her hunger, her energy over the preceding few months, and instead of seeing the ebbing times – low energy, hunger, heightened emotions – as a negative, she could see them as a gift.

From this new space where she felt safe to feel truly embodied, she was able to see these changes in her body, including pain when she felt it, as a signal that her body was functioning or that her nervous system was sending her little messages about her degree of safety. Eva wanted to have a pelvic scan to see if she was ovulating. As crazy as it might sound to you if you're still in the midst of seeing your body as the enemy, Eva was delighting in discovering her body almost as if for the first time.

The connection and joy of true healing

The amazing thing is that when you can take yourself back to that place of safety and regulation in your nervous system, you can be open, present and curious – and the *suffering* of chronic pain can't live in this place. This is the power of holistic physiotherapy as part of a team approach that puts your nervous system state at the heart of healing.

Chapter summary

- Pelvic floor tension is a very common cause of chronic pelvic pain.
- Pelvic floor tension is often a sign that the nervous system is holding on to previous trauma, fear of pain or ongoing stress.
- Tension in the pelvic floor is a protective response. It's important to recognise this, thank your body and then remind it that it is now safe. When we move towards pain without protection, pain is less likely to persist.
- Pelvic floor therapy with a trauma-informed therapist can be an incredibly important part of connecting with your body, finding safety and coming to a place of true healing.

Part 3

Transcendence

16

Connection, meaning and pleasure

We've spoken a lot about pain and how it thrives in a body carrying trauma from the past. We have broken it down into bite-sized pieces so that we can see it for what it is. When we can understand how pain came to be part of us and turn towards it rather than calling it our enemy and trying to fight it or outrun it, it loses the power it held over us. When we are no longer at war with pain, we are no longer at war with our own body and mind. We are liberated.

The path to liberation involves understanding your whole body, your environment and how you exist within our culture. I know that while all this information and the tools we've discussed may bring you hope that things can be different for you and put you on the path to healing, it can also feel overwhelming. Most women living with pelvic pain have been disempowered and feeling hopeless for so long that to hear they have held the power to heal themselves the whole time can feel daunting or confronting. This is where connecting to your team comes in.

None of us can heal alone. We need a community to hold us and provide that sense of safety and stability that's so important as a first step in processing trauma and, I would argue, in healing from chronic pain, because it, too, is characterised by feeling unsafe in your body.

What to look for in a healing team

First and foremost, you want to find a team that listens to your story and treats all of you – not just your pain and definitely not just endometriosis. You also want to find a team of people who make you feel safe – that is, they co-regulate your nervous system and provide a safe and stable place from which to heal. This means that they are trauma-informed, and that they empower you by giving you all the pros and cons of treatment so that you can make an informed decision that is right for you and your body. They don't tell you what to do and they don't speak the language of fear.

Your team of healthcare professionals

You want to find a **doctor** who can talk about the effect of your nervous system and brain on chronic pain, and who addresses gut health and immune system health as part of that. If you're seeing a surgeon who is only interested in surgery or hormonal drugs to 'fight endo', make sure they can talk you through the facts about how likely surgery is to be helpful for you and that they give you all the information regarding potential side effects when it comes to hormonal treatments. If you do decide on surgery, make sure the surgeon is an endometriosis excision specialist, and if they can't talk you through all the other components of pain, make sure they refer you to someone who can.

Many women will need a qualified women's health **pelvic floor physiotherapist** to help guide their body back to safety and teach their body to send messages of safety to the brain, dialling down pain. In my practice this is one of the most helpful parts of therapy.

If you've identified unresolved trauma as part of your story, you might want to work with a **trauma therapist**. Look for one who includes your body and nervous system as part of treatment.

If gut health and bloating are a big part of your story, seeing a **dietician** who can guide you through the best way to nourish your body may be part of your treatment plan as well. But remember that gut health is massively affected by your nervous system state and stress, so if they are a non-diet dietician who can guide you from a place of less restriction and through the lens of polyvagal theory, even better.

This may sound like a lot. Many women with chronic pelvic pain feel like managing their condition is like a full-time job – without the pay and only the cost. I understand that. As the system currently stands, many women need to access these services in the private sector if they want to see someone they choose and without a lengthy wait. The evidence that pelvic pain is best managed in a multidisciplinary team is there – it just needs to be made accessible for every woman early so that she doesn't end up floundering on a 12-month public hospital waiting list.

If you can access these services, remember that it's not a forever process. Caring, trauma-informed and effective practitioners aim to not keep you reliant on them forever but to teach you the tools that will help you live your best life. It might be a journey, but learning these skills will have much longer-lasting results for pain and help improve your health over the long term, which is often far more sustainable financially, physically and emotionally than repeat surgery.

Family and community

As well as a professional team, you want to be able to feel safe to have your needs met by your **family, friends and work** – so talking about what you're going through and asking for support when you need it is really important. Connecting to other **women in your community**, speaking the language of cycles, and encouraging one another to tune in to where you are hormonally so you can give your bodies what they need, is how you start to live in a more aligned way as a woman. For many women, finding a safe **peer support group** where they can tell their story and have their shared experience validated is an important part of healing. Especially if that community aims to elevate women, promotes a positive relationship between women and their body, helps with tools for healing, and helps you live a joyful and meaningful life.

There are lots of support and advocacy groups for endometriosis in Australia that provide encouragement, connection and purpose for many women suffering with pelvic pain. These groups have been vital in sharing women's often untold stories and shining a spotlight on the pain and suffering that in the past women often experienced alone. They have also been platforms for raising awareness of endometriosis and pelvic pain, and for getting much needed government attention and increased funding for services and research into women's health.

We owe a lot to these impressive grassroots women-led movements that have done so much to support women and make it possible for them to share their stories. But I think it's also important to remember that you're so much more than your pain or your endometriosis. While these groups can act as a lifeline for many women who are disconnected and despairing, and while often endometriosis can become a motivating force, purpose or means of connection for many, I want you to remember that healing means coming back to a state of wholeness and not needing to wholly identify with pain or illness.

I've seen many women become stuck in the life of being sick because it provides a valid source of connection and shared vulnerability in a culture that's often devoid of this. It's hugely important to have peer support, access to help and tools, and to know you're not alone. But it's also an important part of healing to remember who you are outside of pain and what it's like to follow your joy. Bonding over shared pain can be therapeutic, but you don't want to live there. There's more to you than your pain.

Out of pain and into joy

I often ask my patients: 'Who are you and what does your life look like without your pain?' Your own answer to this question might give you an idea of what makes your soul sing, what's important to you, what brings joy and meaning to your life. If you can't even imagine what your life would be without pain – which is also common among my patients – start with what brought you joy or pleasure in the past.

When you're in pain and/or stuck in a survival state, finding joy or experiencing pleasure can feel impossible – especially when all your energy goes into trying to ignore or fight pain. It can feel like you're fighting an uphill battle, where there's no room to experience lightness, connection or joy. I want to dispel that myth. We live in an 'and' universe not an 'or' universe. Just as the mind and body cannot be separated and both influence our state of wellness at any given time, so too can pain and pleasure co-exist. A huge part of treatment is simply to remember this and try to tune in to micro-moments of pleasure, connection or joy every day. It's a crucial part of retraining the nervous system back to safety.

Glimmers

Deb Dana, a clinical social worker specialising in polyvagal theory and complex trauma, talks about 'glimmers'. Glimmers are small moments that spark joy and that can help cue the nervous system to feel safe or calm. Whereas triggers send your body into a survival state where pain and protection are more likely, glimmers can bit by bit take you back to safety. That's not to say, if you suffer with chronic pain, that you should find ease and happiness just like that – that's often unrealistic, as you know. The idea is to notice micro-moments of peace even within a hard day or a pain flare.

Noticing these tiny moments of happiness – the smile on the face of a stranger, the purr of your cat, the wag of your dog's tail, sunlight falling through the trees, the smell of rain on asphalt, or the water falling on your back as you shower – can calm your nervous system over time. Each time you notice a glimmer, your brain gets a hit of dopamine and you begin to tether back to your ventral vagal state. Finding more moments of safety leads to more positive feelings and less fear, which can reduce anxiety and stress, and start to retrain your body to feel safe. Increasingly, your body becomes a place where it's harder for chronic pain to live.

When you start noticing glimmers and experiencing their positive effects on your nervous system, you start to look for more, which carves out more roads to safety over time. Even in the midst of pain, your brain is capable of tuning in to positive or neutral sensations. Start by looking for micro-moments of joy and see where it leads you. Remember, pain and pleasure can co-exist if you're aware of it. You can experience pain and simultaneously experience the pleasant sensation of the breath or the sound of calming music. The sensation that grows is the one we pay more attention to.

Exercise: Finding glimmers

Today, set your sights on finding three glimmers. When you notice a glimmer, delight in finding it and savour it. Some people even find it helpful to start a glimmer journal, which is a bit like a gratitude journal. Noticing the sensations you find pleasure in, over time, might lead to even larger chunks of joy. You might even discover what makes your soul sing and start practising it.

1.

....

....

2.

....

....

3.

....

....

Joy and flow

Joy and play, pleasure and connection are vital pieces of the health jigsaw puzzle and a crucial part of my holistic prescription for pain. They're also the first things to fall by the wayside when we become adults, especially if we're living with pain.

Like glimmers, finding what brings you a sense of joy or brings you into a flow state, prioritising it in your life and preferably doing it with others for that ever-important sense of connection, is incredibly helpful in finding your way back to safety in your nervous system. Safety is where joy, play and connection live, and practising joy strengthens our vagal tone, reduces stress and fear, and retrains our nervous system away from pain.

Exercise: Finding what makes your soul sing

This could be something you used to do as a kid, something you've always wanted to try, or something you know you love and lose yourself in. Choose an activity that leaves you feeling calm, connected and invigorated, or one that challenges you and takes you out of your normal life. Or you might do several things. Some ideas include painting, walking in nature, writing, dancing, yoga, sport, baking, gardening, singing, or signing up to play a team sport. My things are pole dancing, yoga, girlfriends, nature and reading novels.

Write down what comes to mind and think about how you can incorporate it into your life on a regular basis.

....

....

....

....

....

....

....

A life of joy is within your reach

Schedule the activity that makes your soul sing, just as you would a doctor's appointment. Finding your joy is probably going to be more health-giving than another health appointment anyway. When you think about it, the aim of healthcare is to get you living a life filled with meaning, love and joy. When you realise that joyful things are still possible even when you experience pain, you're already further along the path to healing than you thought.

Chapter summary

- Healing from chronic pelvic pain is possible and starts when you learn to feel safe in your body again.
- Pay attention to 'glimmers' to help train your nervous system back to safety and joy.
- A multidisciplinary team approach is proven to be helpful to women with chronic pelvic pain.
- Make time to connect to a community that is focused on joy rather than pain.
- There is more to you than pain. Find, or remember, what makes your soul sing and schedule it like a doctor's appointment (it will probably be more beneficial).

17

Rewriting the narrative about periods and our bodies

Changing the paradigm starts with educating women about what's magnificent about their body, teaching them how to listen to what their body is trying to tell them, and learning ways to nurture their body that are based in love and not fear.

As you now know, with your strong understanding of pain through the lens of modern pain science and neurobiology, pain needs fear to grow. Earlier in the book, you also took your first step towards healing, when you learned the truth about what's happening in your body throughout the month. With that, you began to teach your brain to reinterpret your bodily sensations through a lens of safety and even reverence and gratitude rather than fear.

As we have discussed, in our society the menstrual cycle is feared, dismissed or viewed as an inconvenience. This is a mistake, because it sets women up for rejection of their own body and self from an early age. Imagine if women could accept and love themselves in their entirety. Just think how much that would change their experience, their physiology and the world. We don't have time to wait for the wide sweeping change we need in our families, education and medical systems, and society at large. So it has to be up to us to make room and create reverence for women, their bodies and their experiences in the world, so that we can decrease the suffering of women with pain. Change begins one person at a time. I'm hopeful that this book will remind you of the wisdom you already carry in your bones, and the knowledge of the ancient power women have always held. For too long it's been not only hidden, but suppressed and taken from us.

Taking back our power

I'm insanely passionate about teaching girls and women to remember the power they have, and hand back the power that was taken from them thousands of years ago. If women understood their bodies, there would be much less need for medical intervention, much less fear and much less suffering.

When I started practising root-cause medicine, rather than the band-aid solution of treating symptoms that I had been taught, every consultation I had would involve explaining the menstrual cycle and how it's affected by the totality of the woman. I discovered, all too often, that 45-year-old women would have no idea about the changes going on inside them every month and knew even less about the ways their internal hormonal landscape could affect and be affected by their external world. Women were often on the Pill for most of their reproductive lives, many experiencing side effects such as depression and mood disturbance, sexual dysfunction or hair loss, with no idea that these issues could be linked to the Pill.

Several years ago, frustrated over the dearth of knowledge women had about their own bodies, I had the idea of running an educational event for women and girls to explain the menstrual cycle and hormones, and to present non-hormonal ideas for treating common menstrual issues and lifestyle hacks to optimise women's experience in the world. I was inspired by the work of the phenomenal Lucy Peach – an educator and artist who created the award-winning show *The Power of the Period*. In the show, Lucy and her husband, Richard, take the audience through each phase of the menstrual cycle, explaining the four distinct hormonal phases and illuminating the link between our hormonal ebbs and flows and our experience of the world. I thought that if we could combine Lucy's entertaining but accurate and beautiful show with a talk from a gynaecologist, we could empower women so that when things happened in their body they didn't immediately think it was a problem or think their only option was the Pill. Importantly, if they did choose the Pill, I first wanted them to have all the information they needed to make an informed decision, rather than end up on a drug they didn't really understand for the next 20 years.

I thought this was an awesome idea for amplifying what I was trying to do one person at a time in my consultations. At this time, as I was working in a group practice as an associate, I went to the mostly male board for permission to run it as an organisational event. After I pitched my idea at the head of the boardroom table, I was met with a less than enthusiastic response. It seemed that 'health literacy and education' weren't seen as core business and apparently too financially risky to go all in on with me (although they were one of the event's sponsors in the end). I remember the feeling of having my very excited bubble burst.

My first feeling was shame – because I had believed in the value of the idea and knew it to be important but didn't get the validation and approval that I, like so many of us, had been conditioned to seek. My second feeling after driving home in tears was anger. Why did I, a woman, an advocate for women and a highly trained women's health professional, feel that I needed to ask permission from a group of men to help educate and empower women in the first place? This wasn't a slight on the men involved but a reflection on my own sense of powerlessness due to all my good–girl conditioning.

I called my friend and colleague, Elysia Humphries, a naturo-path and former literal rock star who had just had her second baby, and she said: 'Screw it. We can do it ourselves. Let's do it together.' And we did. In six weeks we organised two events, one for women and one for young girls on the cusp of puberty and their parents. More than 600 women and girls attended over two days, and we managed to make $10,000 for a women's charity. It was a success because women are hungry to know themselves.

I will never forget Lucy singing on stage to a group of pre-teen girls a song entitled 'Your Blood Is Amazing' from her EP *Blood Magic*. They looked at her in awe, so proud that they were about to be initiated into this incredible club of womanhood. I felt chills, because I'd never seen the excitement and pride in the eyes of girls and young women when it came to their bodies that I saw in that room that day.

Lucy's lyrics still give me chills:

How can it be that
Nobody told me
What was written into my bones?
Maybe I've always known

For far too long
The treasure has been untold
Worse, it's been told wrong

Your blood is amazing
Your body divine
You can start again every time
It's amazing the moon by your side
You can start again

So much is spilt
So many killed
And we turn and look away

This blood, this body, it's all I have
It's the only way
I can atone for this madness
This mother loving sadness
Your blood is amazing, your body divine

It's not a shame, or even worse
Not a waste
Not a curse

And I can't stand to see your worth
Dripping wasted to the dirt

It's not a secret
(Every laugh and cry, every howl and moan)

I won't keep it
(Every step and stride, buried in your bones)

To myself
Anymore

Lucy's song lyrics convey the pain so many women feel, probably on a subconscious level, about the beauty of our suppressed and hidden inner nature. The opposite is the typical approach in Western society – girls are taught the mechanics of how to manage the inevitably inconvenient period so that it doesn't 'interfere' with their lives, but hardly anything about how to nurture and love themselves over the course of their entire cycle. Seeing those girls swelling with pride as they watched this incredible, strong, proud and beautiful woman singing to them about the magnitude of their superpowers was so moving. In that moment I could see the power of uncovering the truth and providing positive and affirming education. Lucy has since written an amazing book called *Period Queen* that builds on the message of her show. I thoroughly recommend it to any parent of a girl or anyone for that matter, who wants to learn more about the totality of the female body and menstrual cycle. As Lucy says, the menstrual cycle is so much more than just a period.

Ignoring our biology is not equality

Women like Lucy are part of a new movement that not only aims to bring awareness of the experience of having a menstrual cycle into our culture but is also empowering girls and women to be proud of their bodies, talk openly about what they are feeling without shame, and teaching them to ask for what they need to nurture their bodies. For too long we've just learned to use a tampon and get on with it. And we've imbibed the lesson that if we can't just get on with it there's something wrong with us that might need the Pill or an operation. For many women this can help. But what about turning the spotlight on what's wrong with our culture that sets women up to suffer? Perhaps it's not the intrinsic pathology of our bodies that makes us unable to cope with the culture we're trying to fit into, but the culture itself.

It's almost as if, in our quest to be treated as equal to men, we've lost sight of the very real biological fact that our bodies are different. Equality shouldn't be about being treated the same as men – because if we continue to strive for that, we're feeding into the concept of gender bias by constantly measuring ourselves again the 'male standard'. It's not a weakness that we create an egg each month, that our hormones rise and fall in a fashion that's different from men, that our bodies are capable of creating and holding life, or that our bodies have the power to release our uterine lining to start again each month. This difference doesn't make women weak. It makes us bloody amazing.

The idea of the period as a curse still lives on among women in our culture. Cultural anthropologist, Alma Gottlieb, in her essay 'Menstrual Taboos: Moving Beyond the Curse' cites a 1995 study showing that up to 50 per cent of Western women still referred to their period as 'the curse'. She writes: 'the menstrual lessons of Genesis and Leviticus have cast a wide shadow across both time and space . . . With the notion of a curse come specific behaviors and practices that, typically, communities require and women internalize.'

So superimposed upon centuries-old embedded ideas about the inherent shame and wrongness of our bodies, we have a society now that is happy to talk about periods – but only if it doesn't disrupt the capitalistic, patriarchal fabric of our society, and we have an incredibly outdated medical model that reduces women's pain to pelvic lesions, perpetuates fear and further reinforces the idea that there's something fundamentally dangerous going on inside our bodies. If we go back to neuroscience and the concept of predictive coding (where our brain takes shortcuts by influencing our perception of an event or sensation before we actually sense it), it's clear why all this cultural conditioning leads to many women experiencing more pain.

This means that if we're told our periods will be painful, if we expect they will be hard because our culture forces us to push through, and if we think that if they're painful then we have a terrible disease, our brain will be more likely to 'predict and produce pain' – even if the actual sensory input from our body isn't sending a danger signal. It's an error in the way we process information and make sense of the world from that top-down or brain-derived place. This is why it's so important to become embodied, and quiet and still enough to actually feel our sensations.

When we look at our cultural conditioning and how it affects the brain, we can see why our attitudes about our periods will affect our experience of our period. The evidence backs this up: girls with a more positive attitude towards their period generally experience fewer symptoms. This is why women like Lucy Peach, who are helping to rewrite the stories we are told about our bodies and periods, are so important in changing our brains. If we make a positive association with what a period means – that our body has made our hormones that month, which helps with health on every level (not just our ability to have a baby if we want to) – *and* we live in a society that gives women time and space to nurture their body without guilt or shame, our brains might predict something entirely different.

Our stress levels might also be lower, which can reduce inflammation and relieve pelvic floor muscle tension. The simple truth is that living in a culture that allowed us to be as we are and revered our bodies for their difference would take away the trauma of living in a world that isn't made for us. We might feel loved and nurtured by our culture and hence develop a more loving, nurturing relationship with ourselves.

Watch your language

The power of language is incredibly important when it comes to how we think about our body. Words hold power and they can get stuck in our consciousness even over thousands of years – just think about how many women, even recently, have referred to their periods as a curse and just how that affects how we process the experience of a period.

You are not your pain, and you are not your trauma, but they are part of the story of your life. You can see how carrying trauma and being unaware of the effects it may be having on your physical body and brain can cut you off from your body, dialling up your internal warning system and all your protective mechanisms, and how the constant unconscious threat of danger makes you feel like you're fighting an enemy within. In the standard approach to treating pelvic pain you can see how searching for an 'enemy' like endometriosis makes sense.

But if you have endometriosis, it's not separate from you; it's cells in your body like the rest of your cells. And as we've seen, most of the time pain is not down to the endometriosis lesions but to those dialled-up pain pathways and a dysregulated nervous system. Continuing to call these symptoms 'endo' pain or 'endo symptoms' stops you getting to the root of what's actually happening in your body and keeps you focused on fighting an enemy within – both of which increase pain by increasing fear. Using language that conveys the idea of being at war with a part of yourself – such as 'endo-warrior' or 'fighting' or 'enemy' – tells your brain that you are indeed in danger.

When we learn to listen with curiosity rather than fear, through an informed lens of modern pain science and with a nervous system that feels safe, pain stops becoming our enemy and becomes something we can observe and learn from. The good news is that just in the way negative language affects the brain and our experience, so too does using positive language.

Calm birthing or hypnobirthing both aim to use gentle and sensitive language when working with couples as they birth their babies. It has been shown that using words such as 'surge' rather than 'contraction' and 'tension' rather than 'pain', can have a profound impact on the experience and outcome of giving birth. Words like 'pain' and 'contraction' can create more stress, more muscle tension and more pain, which reduces the quality of the birth and can even alter its outcome. In the same way, using phrases such as 'ruptured cyst' to describe the process of ovulation can provoke more fear and more pain. We don't just need to ensure that women understand what's happening inside them each month, we need to use positive and affirming language as we do so.

It's important to start helping our young girls understand this from an early age so that they feel more excited than fearful about getting their first period. How we prepare our girls matters so much, because if they start highly stressed or expecting pain, it's more likely that this is what they'll get.

Womanhood is a gift to celebrate

The greatest gift we can give ourselves is the gift of knowledge and reconnection to our inner guidance system. Not only will this help us live healthier lives with less pain, hormonal havoc and fertility issues, but it will give us courage to live in a way that's in harmony with the rhythm of our body and not against it. Understanding how our body changes throughout our menstrual cycle, appreciating why we're different at different phases, and learning to love ourselves in every phase is the path to becoming fully embodied, bold and powerful women who are proud of who we are in every single cell of our body.

We are not monophasic creatures, and becoming fluent in the language of our cycle will not only help us uncover optimal health, fertility and a greater sense of ease, but is the actual key to living a fully connected and truly authentic life. This is what I wish every woman knew. It seems crazy to think that understanding the ancient rhythms of our body and how we can use this knowledge to our advantage in this modern world is a radical act. But it is, because through our conditioning, even we believe that our female bodies are constantly betraying us. The whole world is built for someone with a 24-hour hormonal cycle (i.e. men), and everything in our culture tells us that the only way we can succeed is to change and mould ourselves to fit a system that was never designed for us.

This is where we start redesigning the world to fit us too.

When women are no longer living out of alignment with their true essence and when Yin energy holds a place just as powerful as Yang energy, the world will be a more beautiful place for everyone. That's how something as simple as understanding and living with our hormonal rhythms can be so radically life-changing.

If you need a refresher as to just how amazing our bodies are, turn back to Chapter 1 and read the description of a normal period again. Remind yourself just how amazing you are, and just what a miracle your body is.

It starts with the knowledge.
Knowledge brings power.
Power brings change.

18

Embracing our period as a time for radical self-care

I hope that now you understand just how incredible your internal symphony is every month, and that a period is actually the sign that you've matured and released an egg and made a cocktail of hormones essential to the health of your whole body, you can start to see your cycle in a new light. It's not an annoying accident of biology; it gives us the opportunity to start again every month. Women are in the unique position of cycling through creation and destruction and letting go every month. No one season of the year is better than the others – they are just different. No one part of your cycle is better or worse than another. When the leaves fall off the trees and winter comes, we can see the beauty of the natural world and the meaning behind the cycles of growth and falling away. We need to learn to see the same beauty reflected inside us. We do different things in winter as opposed to summer – we might spend more time indoors, cuddle up, create more cosiness and nurturing. We can apply the same lessons to our internal winter – our period.

People such as Lucy Peach and other menstrual cycle educators are already showing you the way. Not only does Lucy speak about all the phases of the menstrual cycle, she talks about *feeling* your way into your body and what it needs throughout each phase. She describes the period phase as the 'dream' phase or winter – a quiet time to rest, regroup and prepare for the cycle ahead. The period is nature's pit stop, and when we start to see it as an inevitable and beautiful part of the cyclical nature of the female body, we give ourselves permission to feel our way into our own unique body's needs when we're bleeding.

Making our periods a time of self-care

Imagine a world where instead of something to be feared, ashamed of or just annoyed by, your period was that time once a month when you stopped, connected inwards and gave your body what it needs. How would thinking about your period as the ultimate self-care part of the month change how you view or anticipate it?

It might be that you carry on as normal but plan for that time in your cycle by giving yourself a break – ordering in, cooking meals in advance, having a long bath, booking a massage or a gentle yoga class after work. If you have more challenging periods, it might mean that you plan to take a day off work or study from home on that day. Just the change of being in a safe space where you can move, rest and be, with more freedom and spaciousness to care for yourself, can take the pressure off, reduce pain and flip the experience of your period on its head. I've seen first-hand the huge improvement in quality of life and pain reduction that comes when we give women permission to take their power back and create the space to nurture themselves.

This is the time to connect with yourself. Journal on what has served you in the past month and what you dream for the month ahead. Traditionally, menstruation was seen as a time when a woman had deeper access to her own wisdom and intuition, so use it to connect to what's true for you. Slowing down and creating space for yourself here, and in the week before, honours your wise woman. If you rush past, pretending it's not happening or dreading it, there is no space to honour her. This is especially true if your period is painful – your body is asking you to rest more, to meet yourself where you are. To nurture yourself.

Connect with the loves in your life. Allow yourself to be cared for. Accept the hugs, the cups of tea and the home-cooked meals. If you're like most women, you care for everyone else all month long. This is your chance to be looked after, and it starts with your own nurturing and self-compassion. If *you* can't look after you, how can you expect anyone else to?

Right now, this very phase, start practising. It might look like a long bath after work, essential oils, self-massage, a facial, self-pleasure. It's true – orgasm helps with cramping and is the ultimate self-love practice. Now is the time for rest and care. If we could redefine winter as a time of rest and restoration, we would almost look forward to this time rather than be conditioned to loathe it. Can you imagine a world where women were revered during their period? Where they were celebrated, nourished and allowed to rest? I can. There would be a whole lot less women in my clinic if the world gave women the space, time and recognition they deserve. It starts with us giving the time to ourselves and honouring our own body and the wise woman who lives inside us and remembers our power. We can only hope the world follows.

The basics of period self-care

During week 1 of your cycle – your period – aim to:

Do more	Do less
Resting and dreaming	High-intensity exercise
Gentle movement	Looking after every everyone else
Eating of warming, easy-to-digest foods	Eating of spicy foods and raw cold foods
Spending time in nature	Looking at devices and other technology

Exercise: Plan your radical self-care day

Using the ideas above or your own, think about how you could reframe your period* as time for radical self-care. Think about the things that soothe you, that bring you comfort and joy, and start planning for your next period so everything is in place.

If you need to organise a day off, do it now. Book a massage. Ask someone to cook for you or have meals in the freezer ready to go. See if you can feel your way into the idea of planning something 'pleasurable' for this part of your cycle. Remember, you can have discomfort or pain and experience pleasure at the same time – but you need to be relaxed, connected and embodied to get there. This is why a regular rest and embodiment practice is so important.

If you do experience pain, make sure you have your pain flare plan (see pages 276–81) somewhere you can easily access it. It's also a good idea to make a list of all the things that soothe your nervous system and widen your window of tolerance – go back to Chapter 12 for ideas.

Journal about your perfect self-care day and start anticipating it. Ask yourself how it feels in your body to think of planning your period in this way rather than through the lens of fear.

Journal prompts for self-care

- *What can I let go of that no longer serves my highest good?*

....

....

- *What are my dreams for the month ahead?*

....

....

- *What worked for me this month?*

....

....

- *What didn't work this month?*

....

....

- *How can I soothe my nervous system during this time?*

....

....

- *How can I practise more self-compassion?*

....

....

- *How can I practise giving my body what it needs right now?*

....

....

- *How can I meet myself where I am?*

....

....

- *How can I experience pleasure in my body even when I experience pain?*

....

....

- *If I experience pain how can I soften into it and listen rather than go into protection mode?*

....

....

If you don't get periods because you're on the Pill continuously, your periods are suppressed through other hormonal means, you don't have a uterus or you've gone through menopause, still plan a self-care day once a month. You can use the phases of the moon as a prompt if that feels right for you. The value of rest is horribly underestimated in our culture, and having a regular time to just be at least once a month (but preferably for some moments every day) is highly conducive to reducing the stress and pressures of modern life.

Exercise: Yoga and meditation for your period

Yoga is an amazing way to connect with ourselves and feel our way into our body when we spend so much time in our head and living a life that doesn't support our physical body. Week 1 is the perfect time to use yoga to nourish ourselves. You don't need to fit in a class or go anywhere special; you just need a few minutes, a mat or a soft surface, and a desire to feel truly embodied. Try these (pelvic floor physiotherapist-approved) poses during your period to relieve cramps and help ground yourself in your body.

Cat/cow pose
Starting on all-fours, inhale as you gently drop your belly and exhale as you arch your back. Do several rounds to mobilise your hips and relieve tension around the pelvis. Hold any position that feels good and what your body needs at the time.

Cobra pose
Lie on your belly with your hands beneath your shoulders and your elbows by your sides. Press your hands into the floor and tighten your bottom, arching your back up and keeping your feet as close together as you can. Stretch your neck and look up towards the ceiling, aiming to hold for one minute with long deep breathing. This pose massages your ovaries and uterus and stretches the muscles around your spine.

Locust pose
Lie on your belly with your hands in fists just under your hips. Press your heels together and keep your chin on the floor. With your legs straight and your shoulders relaxed, raise your legs off the

floor (it may not be very high) and hold with deep breathing for up to one to two minutes. This is a strengthening lower-back stretch.

Legs up the wall
Lie on the floor with your legs at 90 degrees up a wall, take long deep breaths into your belly, then relax completely onto your mat. This pose helps strengthen the back and abdominal muscles and can aid with detoxification and digestion.

Child's pose
Starting on all-fours with your knees slightly wider than hip-width apart, lower your hips towards your heels as you lean forward, extending your arms in front of you. Allow your torso to relax and sink down towards the mat. You can keep your arms extended or bring them back alongside your body – whichever feels more comfortable. Focus on deep, gentle breaths, allowing your body to relax and release tension. This can help alleviate any discomfort or pressure on the abdomen, while still providing a soothing and restorative posture during menstruation.

Remember, it's essential to listen to your body and modify or skip any poses that don't feel right for you during this time

Exercise: Reflect on your radical self-care day
Journal on your self-care experience using these prompts.

How did it feel to give yourself permission to rest and set yourself up in a comfortable space rather than pushing through?

....

....

....

Were you able to manage your period any differently?

....

....

....

Were you able to find any glimmers of joy or pleasure?

....

....

What would you do differently next time to create an even more nurturing experience?

....

....

A brave and wonderful new world

I can envisage a utopia where women's bodies are not forced to fit into the male standard. There is even evidence that in many facets of society we are heading in the right direction – such as menstrual leave being granted in some countries and even in some workplaces in Australia. But we still have a long way to go. While we need to continue to push for wider societal change, I strongly believe that we don't have to wait for that change to happen.

Change starts with us right now and the way we view our body. When we understand how remarkable we are, we can take steps right away to rewrite the meaning of menstruation in our own life and in the communities of women around us. There are lots of things we do have the power to change, and we don't have to ask for or wait for permission to nurture ourselves. We can simply take back our power and step into that embodied version of ourselves we've always been.

Many people say this is unrealistic and things like menstrual leave would bring businesses and the economy to their knees. Maybe that's what's needed – less focus on productivity at all costs and more focus on a sustainable society that honours women in the way it should be honouring the earth. Women are not a minority. We're talking about changing the way we treat 50 per cent of the world's humanity. The world is set up to fit the bodies of men, but that's no reason why it shouldn't be able to make room for women.

I know it seems radical to suggest that slowing down and caring for ourselves might be helpful – because we've been conditioned to believe that success is go, go, go and more, more, more and do, do, do.

I hope you're getting angry. I hope you're angry that our Western culture has instilled in us a fear and loathing of our bodies down to our very bones. I hope you're angry that the pain of carrying that internalised hatred has been reduced only to endometriosis, forcing many women without that diagnosis to turn on themselves still further. When we fight against a part of us that we've labelled bad or evil, we allow danger and fear to persist, which drives pain. For most women with pelvic pain, the real problem is their environment, their nervous system and how our culture sets us up to experience more pain.

Perhaps anger isn't going to get us anywhere either. Perhaps what we need is radical love for ourselves. Enough love to reject the idea that to be a woman is to suffer, that it's our lot in life. Enough love to reject society dismissing women's power and making us think we're empowered only if we can ignore our own biology. We need to reject the culture and not ourselves. When we women can take up the space of reverence in the world that was always ours, remember just how incredible our bodies truly are, and create a world that fits us rather than trying to squeeze into something that was never designed for us, we will truly be empowered. And I bet there would be far fewer women experiencing chronic pain.

It takes great courage to lean in to our female bodies, listen to them and act in alignment with what they're asking of us when everything in the outside world is pulling us in another direction.

It really is a radical act to honour our unique hormonal cycle and ask the external world to rise up and meet us where we are. But that's what we must do if we are to evolve into fully embodied women. We are multidimensional goddesses, and if we can honour and love ourselves there will be no stopping us.

Jess's pain story, part 3

Jess's history with pain and with trauma was very complex, but she has managed to come a long way since I first met her.

She continues to be supported by her psychiatrist and pain specialist, but began seeing our physiotherapists, Angie and Brooke, to help with recognising the link between a flare and pelvic floor tension.

We have done some pain reprocessing therapy and lots of yoga under our big tree at Vera and spend lots of time helping Jess to find safety in her body. Jess is now off the Pill and having manageable periods without the need to use opiates. She has spent time with a trauma therapist and a life coach and has been able to focus on her life and what she wants out of it, rather than focusing on her pain.

Jess still has some pain, but it doesn't consume her like it used to and she is able to make time to care for herself during her period, and no longer finds them a dreadful part of her month. In fact, her pain is now less than when she was on hormonal drugs to suppress her bleeding because of her understanding about her nervous system and pain pathways. Most of all, Jess has felt supported by her team and in doing so has been able to learn about and support herself so much more.

Chapter summary

- Menstrual cycle education, support and space to nurture your body all improve your experience of your period.
- Taking the time to honour your body when you have your period rather than pushing through, can reduce stress, tension and pain.
- It's time to redefine your period as a time to tune into your body, listen and give it what it needs. The revolution starts with you!

Conclusion:
A new paradigm for pelvic pain care

You have probably picked this book up because either you or someone you love has been suffering with chronic pelvic pain and are anywhere between frustrated and deeply despairing about the current treatment options.

Persistent pelvic or period pain can be deeply distressing and it's easy to feel stuck and as if there is no way out. Some women feel like pain controls their entire life, making joy, pleasure or connection impossible. If you've been diagnosed with endometriosis you may feel the weight of an incurable chronic disease and that the only options you have are repeated surgeries, hysterectomy or hormonal medication. And while surgeries and hormones may always be part of a treatment plan for many women, successful treatment always requires a whole-person approach. If you have chronic pelvic pain and don't have endometriosis, you may have been feeling even more lost – because you haven't come across any readily available answers or solutions to your pain.

Having read this book, you now know that chronic pain is far more nuanced than the presence or absence of a 'structural' cause. Most people who have chronic pain will have some evidence of neuroplastic pain or pain system hypersensitivity – meaning the immune system pain pathways and the brain are producing or amplifying pain sensations based on faulty assessments of danger driven by a dysregulated nervous system.

Persistent pelvic pain has its origins in nervous system and immune system dysregulation, which is often precipitated by developmental trauma/chronic stress and the ongoing stressors of our modern lifestyle. Getting to the root of the nervous system dysregulation is the key to allowing the body to function optimally. When we feel safe in our bodies, everything works better and no treatment – drugs, surgery, diet or supplements – will be enough without paying attention to the state of your nervous system which underpins it all.

But through knowledge comes power. Once you understand the bigger picture, you can develop compassion for that amazing body of yours – which is all the time trying to help you survive – and you can learn, with the support of loved ones and experienced professionals, to help it return to a place of safety where it can learn to come back into balance. True and real healing is more than possible.

This process of returning to yourself is about meeting the precious being you are. When you do, you learn to love yourself. From here, real healing can occur. It's possible to find a way out of pain – but by turning towards it rather than away – and this is only possible when we learn to feel safe in our body. You are not your pain and you are not your trauma. But both these things can teach us about your body and help you find more compassion and love for yourself on the path to living a full and meaningful life.

The problem of chronic pelvic pain is not a problem intrinsic to women or explained away by endometriosis. It's also a reflection of a culture that continues to separate the mind and the body, uphold gender biases that don't allow space in society for women and girls to nurture their bodies during their periods, and to pathologise women's bodies when they suffer under the stress of an unsustainable environment.

More than that, it is also a symptom of the failure of governments to address developmental trauma – by undervaluing the role of primary caregivers in society, leading to detachment, neglect and high rates of sexual abuse of young girls and women. These traumas happen in secret and are often chronic and pervasive, increasing not just the risk of pelvic pain but of polycystic ovarian disease, premenstrual dysphoric disorder, and all the other chronic mental and physical illness we know are increased in survivors of childhood trauma.

If you have pelvic pain and trauma – this is not your fault. But you deserve so much better.

My dream is that knowledge of our nervous system and how our experiences shape it will be taught in schools, to parents and from parents to children, alongside all the incredible, simple practices we've used in this book to help us feel regulated when we move into survival mode. Widespread application of this knowledge could halt the potential effects of the impact of chronic stress on the body and prevent all the chronic health conditions, including pain, that we know are linked to developmental trauma. If we simply knew how to care for, befriend and feel compassion for our nervous system, we would gain nervous system flexibility and be able to return to the safe state where our bodies work best.

We need to bring these well-established links between trauma, pain and the role of the brain and nervous system into public consciousness. We need to debunk the myths about endometriosis, which create huge amounts of fear among young women – and fear perpetuates pain. We need to realise that surgery is not the gold standard treatment for chronic pain and is often doing more harm than good.

We need multidisciplinary centres for those who already have persistent pain. But rather than more centres of surgical excellence for endometriosis, our aim should be to prevent the development of persistent pelvic pain in the first place. My vision of a world that really supports women, so they can have a healthy body and a healthy relationship with their pelvis and periods, is this:

- positive and affirming period and menstrual cycle education from a young age.
- a focus on nervous system regulation and the introduction of mindfulness and embodiment therapies in schools and homes. This could look like deep breathing, dancing, doing yoga and laughing together, creating community and allowing co-regulation. Ideally, this shouldn't need to happen in a doctor's office.
- a focus on providing support to caregivers and on establishing strong and healthy parent–child attachments in the early years
- more time for GPs to talk about all the causes of period pain and provide options and solutions that go beyond surgery and hormonal drugs.
- a medical system that recognises that the brain and body are not separate and that treatment of women with chronic pelvic pain needs to take into account the latest research on pain science.
- affordable and accessible physiotherapy, psychology, somatic and embodied therapy, and nutrition therapy, and a system that rewards outcomes rather than number of procedures performed.
- a culture that respects and reveres the differences between men's and women's bodies, and provides time and space for us to care for ourselves during our period in the way that best suits us.

It is my very strong belief that women are the canaries in the coalmine for an unsustainable and sick society. For the vast majority of women, pelvic pain is not just their problem – it points to real problems in the way our culture is set up. We can't change society or culture quickly or obliterate centuries of oppression and shame, but we have the power to choose to live from a place of embodiment rather than bow to the pressures to produce and constantly do. We can choose to be. We can choose to listen to our body and what it's asking of us. We can choose to create and be part of communities that embrace the beauty and cyclical nature of a woman's body. We can choose to nourish and nurture ourselves and give permission for our sisters, our friends, our mothers and, most importantly, our daughters to do the same.

At the risk of sounding very woo-woo, I want to finish with a story from my life. When I was researching this book I was staying in a little country town and went to get a massage. At the end of the massage, my therapist told me she wanted to give me something called the 13th Rite of the Munay Ki – or the rite of the womb. Apparently, the Munay Ki are a series of rites based on the wisdom of the shamans of the Andes and the Amazon. She had no idea that I was a gynaecologist or was writing about pelvic pain.

She placed her hands in the air and said the words:

There is a lineage of women who freed themselves from suffering.
This lineage of women wants us to remember the womb is not a place to store fear and pain.
The womb is to create and give birth to life.

She put her hands on her womb space and repeated the same words:

The womb is not a place to store fear and pain.
The womb is to create and give birth to life.

She placed my hands on my womb space and I repeated the same words:

The womb is not a place to store fear and pain.
The womb is to create and give birth to life.

She told me to share this rite with as many women as possible. So here I am, trying to share it with all of you.

My greatest wish is that women know how incredible, how powerful and how beautiful they are and that without them creation and life wouldn't be possible. A period is simply a reminder of that power. If you have pain or issues with your periods, you do have the power to heal and there are so many options available to you. Understanding your body and its beauty without fear, and why pain and suffering sometimes happen, is a huge step towards healing. Knowing that you are in charge and you get to make the decisions that feel right for you gives you back your power. For some women it's hormones and surgery, for some just hormones, for others a more natural approach, for others still a mixture of all modalities. The important thing is that treatment always addresses the nervous system, the pelvic floor and the immune system – or simply speaking, the whole woman and the culture in which she resides. Only then is true healing possible.

I know there may be some backlash for my position. It is at odds with everything in the public discourse about the importance of early diagnosis of endometriosis and surgery for everyone. But it comes from experience. This book is for the women in my office whose stories I bear witness to. It is my greatest privilege to hold space for these women, their pain, their healing and their transcendence.

Transcendence is possible for you too.

Acknowledgements

To everyone in the Vera community and to my sisters in our quest to help women remember the magic their bodies hold, especially Dr Thea Bowler and Dr Alice Whittaker, for the hundreds of hours of conversation, messages and 3 am book editing. This is your book as much as it is mine – your friendship and support are everything.

To Brooke Dobó and Desi Carlos, for their expertise and contribution to this book.

To Ingrid, Bec, Nicola and the team at Pan Macmillan, who I am so grateful to for helping to send this book out into the world.

To Stephanie Don, for creating amazing graphics from my scribbly pictures and terrible handwriting with a short deadline.

To Lucy Peach, Lara Briden, Susan Evans and everyone out there doing the important work of helping women know and remember their power. You all inspire me and give me the strength to keep going. Together I know we can help change the world for women.

To Ainslee Palmer, whose vulnerability, strength and creativity are a tremendous example that transformation from pain is possible.

And to Rob, Lucia, Richie, Jude and Mum and Dad, for believing in the importance of this work and supporting me and my dream of helping women to find safety in their bodies and their world, every step of the way. It would all be impossible without you.

A pain flare tool kit to bring you back to safety

Adapted from a guide by Associate Professor Susan Evans
(specialist, researcher, educator and advocate in pelvic pain)

Pain flares describe when you have an increase in pain from your usual level. When you understand the common causes for a flare in pain you can bring your body back to a place of safety and get your pain under control.

Causes:

- a period or breakthrough bleeding on hormonal drugs
- pelvic floor muscle spasm
- urinary tract infection
- constipation or IBS
- stress and poor sleep – **often underpins or exacerbates a flare.**

Treatment:

- don't panic – the flare will settle
- keep practising gentle movement – 'freezing' sends a message of danger to your brain, which exacerbates pain and muscle tension leading to more pain
- keep rest times short – less than 30 minutes – before getting up and stretching or moving around
- remember your mantra – 'I'm sore, but I'm safe.'
- adjust medications as needed to manage bleeding, pain or bowel symptoms – but avoid opioids which usually make chronic pain worse
- keep connected with loved ones and your care team.

The Brain: Calming the nervous system from the top (top-down therapy)

- Remember the things that can cause pain during a period and that you are safe and not in danger.
- A great affirmation to calm you down is: 'It's just a flare. I'm sore, but safe. I have a plan.'
- Practise the pain reprocessing exercise on page 212.
- Use deep breathing to come back into the body, allow the pain to be there and notice it without judgement, notice other positive sensations in the body and continue to remind yourself that you are safe.
- Use guided meditation or breathing apps if this is easier – for example, CALM, Headspace, Curable.
- Maintain regular sleep practices – sleep deprivation makes pain worse.
- Co-regulate with safe people in your life.
- Revisit the coming back to safety practices in Chapter 16.

Pelvic floor muscle spasm: Feeling into the body (bottom-up therapy)

- Maintain a practice of gentle movement – preferably in nature, which unlocks the pelvis and core and calms the nervous system. Remember pain on movement does not equal tissue damage – it is safe to move. Pain comes from the desire to freeze and protect.
- Use gentle stretches to relax the pelvis: pelvicpain.org.au/wp-content/uploads/2019/01/Stretches---Women.pdf
- Do gentle yoga, see pages 264–5.
- Practise deep belly breathing.
- Try the body scan exercises and other practices in Chapter 15.

Constipation/IBS flare: Calm the nervous system to allow for optimal digestion

- Gut symptoms can frequently be the result of stress and nervous system dysregulation which can exacerbate existing pain or cause a pain flare.
- If constipated, ensure you are drinking enough water 1.5–2 litres per day.
- Relaxed toileting postures with knees higher than your hips – a relaxed pelvic floor, will also help.
- Gentle stretching and walking will help with bloating.
- Abdominal massage can be helpful.
- Peppermint tea can help to improve digestion.
- Increasing dietary fibre – add some figs or prunes to a high-fibre breakfast, such as oats.
- Use a glycerine suppository from the pharmacy if you're still unable to pass a motion.
- Movicol with a stool softener like lactulose can also help if taken daily until symptoms improve.
- Avoid opioid medications as these will make constipation worse.
- See a doctor if you don't experience any improvement.

Urinary tract infection or painful bladder syndrome

- The bladder can become painful in women with chronic pelvic pain and/or endometriosis due to inflammation of the bladder and pain system hypersensitivity.
- If you think you have a UTI, see a doctor and get appropriate antibiotics as soon as you can.
- Sometimes, because of pain system hypersensitivity, it can feel like you have an infection when there isn't one. In these instances:
  o make sure you empty your bladder regularly
  o use relaxed toileting postures and double void (spend extra time on the toilet to completely empty your bladder)

o dilute and alkalise your urine by drinking 400ml of water mixed with a teaspoon of bicarb soda or one sachet of Ural. You can use a Ural sachet twice daily

o avoid acidic foods and alcohol

o take two paracetamol and an anti-inflammatory medication like ibuprofen

o use your calming top-down and bottom-up techniques.

Period (or breakthrough bleeding) management tool kit

Manage Flow

- Period undies
- Menstrual cups and steriliser
- Tranexamic acid (Cyklokapron) and anti-inflammatory, e.g. Mefenamic acid (Ponstan) to reduce heavy flow:
  o take 2 tablets of each for breakfast, lunch and dinner
  o start as soon as you notice the bleeding and continue for the heavy days – maximum seven days
  o you can also try just one or two of these on heavy days for minor improvement
  o together it will reduce flow by 40 per cent.

Non-pharmacological ways to manage pain

- Stick-on heat packs, hot water bottle, wheat bag
- TENS machine, e.g. Mira Pro: mirapro.com.au
- Gentle yoga, see pages 264–5
- **Pelvic floor pain:**
  o gentle stretches to relax the pelvis: pelvicpain.org.au/wp-content/uploads/2019/01/Stretches---Women.pdf
  o gentle yoga – see pages 264–5
  o deep belly breathing
  o a valium suppository if relaxation exercises are not helpful – these need to be prescribed by your doctor.

Anti-inflammatories (e.g. Ponstan)

- Aim to reduce prostaglandins
- Take one day before period starts, if you can predict
- Take maximum dose on the box, regularly throughout the day
- Always take with food
- Avoid opioids (e.g. panadeine forte, codeine, endone)

Supplements to reduce pain and flow

- Magnesium Glycinate, e.g. Ethical Nutrients Mega Mag – 1 scoop (300mg), all through the month, increasing to 2 scoops during period days
- Fish Oil, e.g. Bioceutical EPA/DHA Ultraclean – 1 to 2 a day, all through the month
- Zinc – 30mg with food, daily; you can get this as part of a multivitamin or a standalone
- Ginger root capsules, e.g. Nature's Sunshine – 500mg, three times a day during period days
- Curcumin, e.g. BioCeuticals Theracurmin Triple – 1 tablet daily
- NAC (N-Acetyl Cysteine) – 600–1200mg per day
- Iron, e.g. Maltofer, and Vitamin C, at night

Don't forget your environment

Know and honour your cycle

- Honour your 'dream' phase or winter – rest and reflect – consider working from home
- Practise deep belly breathing
- Eat warming and nourishing foods and drinks, such as herbal teas
- Have a bath
- Self-massage with essential oils
- Burn a candle and do some journaling
- Tune into pleasure even if you have pain – ask: 'How can I

honour and nurture myself when my body is asking to be cared for? What could feel good right now?'

- Resources:
  - ○ 'Unlocking the power of your cycle' (e-course) by Dr Peta Wright: verawomenswellness.com.au/utpoyc
  - ○ 'The Power of the Period' by Lucy Peach, TEDxPerth: ted.com/talks/lucy_peach_the_power_of_the_period
  - ○ *Period Queen: Life hack your cycle and own your power all month long* by Lucy Peach

A guide to finding the right practitioner

If periods are consistently painful or you are experiencing pelvic pain on most days, and have tried the strategies in this book with no improvement, please see a women's health GP promptly. This is not because of the fear of endometriosis but for you to get some help to manage pain early, which is the most important thing in preventing chronic pain.

At your GP, ask for a good quality TV ultrasound if you are sexually active. If you are not sexually active, a transabdominal ultrasound is a good first step to exclude endometriomas, other ovarian cysts or other acute causes of pain. I would only ask for an MRI if these other strategies have not been successful.

If the result of a good quality ultrasound comes back normal, you can be fairly confident that there is no deep or ovarian endometriosis. You can also be reassured that a laparoscopy is unlikely to uncover much more at this point because, in all likelihood, you may have superficial endometriosis which we know exists almost 50 per cent of the time, and that this regresses or remains the same in 70 per cent of cases, and is least likely to respond well to surgery.

Discuss alternative treatments with your GP, such as hormonal therapy and tranexamic acid.

Your GP can provide you with a care plan and, if asked, they can refer you to a dietician who specialises in gut health and women's health, a trauma-informed pelvic floor physiotherapist or a trauma therapist if this is part of your story.

Pelvic floor physiotherapists

Vera Women's Wellness (QLD): verawomenswellness.com.au/physiotherapy

All Women's Health (QLD): allwomenshealth.com.au

Breathe Health (QLD): breathehealth.com.au

The Healthy Peach Physiotherapy (QLD): thehealthypeachphysio.com.au

Pelviology Physiotherapy (QLD): pelviology.com.au

Pear Exercise Physiology and Physiotherapy (QLD): pearexercisephysiology.com.au

Sue Croft Physiotherapy (QLD): suecroftphysiotherapist.com.au

The Physiotherapy Clinic Sydney (NSW): physiotherapyclinic.com.au

Hawkesbury Family Health collective (NSW): hawkesburyfamilyhealthcollective.com.au

The Studio Rozelle (NSW): thestudiorozelle.com.au

Dubbo Pelvic Health Clinic (NSW): dubbopelvichealthclinic.com.au

Inner North Physiotherapy (VIC): innernorthphysiotherapy.com.au

Ivory Rose Physiotherapy (SA): ivoryrosephysio.com.au

The Pelvic Pain Foundation also has a comprehensive guide of physiotherapists in each state and territory: pelvicpain.org.au

Pain and trauma therapy

Blue Knot Foundation – has lots of resources on trauma therapy and help for finding a therapist.
blueknot.org.au/survivors/finding-support

Natajsa Wagner (QLD) – has a course and a great list of free resources on her website.
natajsawagner.com

Sarah Dakhili (QLD) – has a great podcast and a list of free resources on her website.
mentalawakening.com.au

Pain reprocessing therapists

Note: many pain psychologists will practice similar techniques.

Terry Nelson
Psychologist
Coolum Beach, QLD
jacarandacounselling.com

Sarah Dakhili
Psychotherapist and Mental
Health Social Worker
Wilston, QLD
mentalawakening.com.au

G.E. Poole
Psychologist
Gold Coast, QLD
corehealthcare.com.au/
gold-coast

Kathleen Doyle
Rehabilitation Counsellor
North Manly, NSW
hdtraining.com.au

Lanhowe Chen
Clinical Psychologist
Deakin, ACT
www.painless.health

Don Mackenzie
Accredited Mental Health
Social Worker
Brunswick, VIC
socialsense.com.au

Garth Bennett
Psychologist
Melbourne, VIC
garthbennett.com.au

Geordie Thompson
Hypnotherapist
Perth, WA
hypnologicsolutions.com.au

Other trauma therapists I regularly recommend who have a somatic (body) focus:
Alison Bremner – trauma sensitive yoga therapist
devishaktiyoga.com

Claire Stephensen – somatic and creative arts practitioner
verawomenswellness.com.au/claire-stephensen

Dieticians

Desi Carlos, Tree of Life Nutrition (QLD) – for advice on an anti-inflammatory diet
treeoflifenutrition.com.au

Lisa Carrigg (QLD) – non-diet dietician and intuitive eating coach
verawomenswellness.com.au/lisa-carrigg-dietitian

Referral pathways for surgery – public system

If you need surgery and are going through the public system, don't just wait for surgery – remember, chronic pain is always multifactorial and surgery alone is not effective at addressing all the other factors. If accessible to you, in the interim you can also try hormones, physiotherapy, dietary or trauma therapy.

The Australian Government has recently provided funding for dedicated pelvic pain clinics which may be a good place to start if you need more specialised care than your GP can provide.

Locations of Australian Government-funded Endometriosis and Pelvic Pain GP Clinics			
State / Territory	Successful Clinic	Location	Primary Health Network
NSW	Orange Family Medical Centre	Orange, NSW	Western NSW PHN
	Hunters Hill Medical Practice	Hunters Hill, NSW	Northern Sydney PHN
	Leichhardt General Practice	Leichardt, NSW	Central and Eastern Sydney PHN
	The Women's Health Centre Southern Highlands	Mittagong, NSW	South Western Sydney PHN
	Milton Medical Centre	Milton, NSW	South Eastern NSW PHN
	Coffs Harbour Women's Health Centre	Coffs Harbour, NSW	North Coast PHN
VIC	EACH Practice	Ringwood East, VIC	Eastern Melbourne PHN
	Bendigo Community Health Services	Bendigo, VIC	Murray PHN
	Kardinia Health	Belmont, VIC	Western Victoria PHN
	Lyndoch Medical Hub	Warrnambool, VIC	Western Victoria PHN

State / Territory	Successful Clinic	Location	Primary Health Network
QLD	MATSICHS (Institute for Urban Indigenous Health Ltd)	Morayfield, QLD	Brisbane North PHN
	Benowa Super Clinic	Benowa, QLD	Gold Coast PHN
	True Relationships and Reproductive Health	Cairns, QLD	Northern Queensland PHN
	Neighbourhood Medical	Bardon, QLD	Brisbane North PHN
WA	Pioneer Health Albany	Albany, WA	Country WA PHN
	The Garden Family Medical Clinic	Murdoch, WA	Perth South PHN
SA	Kadina Medical Associates	Kadina, SA	Country SA PHN
TAS	Family Planning Tasmania	Glenorchy, TAS	Tasmania PHN
ACT	Sexual Health and Family Planning ACT (SHFPACT)	Canberra, ACT	ACT PHN
NT	Northside Health Darwin	Coconut Grove, NT	Northern Territory PHN

If you can't access private services, most large public hospitals also have pelvic pain and chronic pain clinics and your GP will be able to refer you there, where you can access psychology, physiotherapy and pain services. By the time this book is published there may also be specialised multidisciplinary endometriosis and pelvic pain clinics in some centres. These clinics do have long waitlists, so remember that there is so much you can do now by following the recommendations in this book and checking out the resource section for more affordable and easy-to-access supports.

Gynaecology and surgery - private system

If you decide to see a private gynaecologist, make sure you see someone who works in a multidisciplinary team or who has a referral network they work closely with.

If you need or decide to have surgery, ensure that your surgeon is an endometriosis excision specialist and has a holistic approach, and that they have a plan that doesn't just involve surgery if your pain returns.

The pelvic pain society has a list of registered practitioners interested in pain: pelvicpain.org.au/find-support/find-a-health-professional

Vera Women's Wellness (verawomenswellness.com.au) is in Queensland and is a private multidisciplinary health clinic that includes gynaecologists, physiotherapists, a GP, psychotherapists, embodiment coaches, a health coach, a naturopath and dieticians.

When choosing a practitioner, ensure they have a solid grasp of the causes of pelvic pain – including causes outside the pelvis and can refer you elsewhere if they do not. Always ensure you have a thorough explanation of the pros and cons of any treatment and that you feel in charge of the direction of your treatment.

Remember that you don't have to wait to change your experience with pain. You have the power to change your nervous system, your diet, your stress levels and your environment. This book will give you the tools to start.

Resources

Australian endometriosis clinical practice guideline
- ranzcog.edu.au/wp-content/uploads/2022/02/Endometriosis-clinical-practice-guideline.pdf

Pelvic Pain Foundation
- pelvicpain.org.au
- Easy stretches to relax the pelvis: pelvicpain.org.au/wp-content/uploads/2019/01/Stretches-%E2%80%93-Women.pdf

Vera Women's Wellness
- verawomenswellness.com.au

Resources for understanding chronic pain

Websites
- Tame the Beast: tamethebeast.org/resources
- 'Why Things Hurt' by Lorimer Moseley, TEDxAdelaide: youtube.com/watch?v=gwd-wLdIHjs
- Understanding pain in less than 5 minutes (Live Active Chiropractic): youtube.com/watch?v=C_3phB93rvI
- The Drug Cabinet in the Brain (Neuro Orthopaedic Institute NOI): youtube.com/watch?v=Gd2NaGZa7M4
- Thought Viruses (Neuro Orthopaedic Institute NOI): youtube.com/watch?v=7eQpRZxXv2g

Rebooting pain programs (online)

- This Way Up: thiswayup.org.au/how-we-can-help/courses/chronic-pain
- Pain Reprocessing Therapy: painreprocessingtherapy.com
- The Cure for Chronic Pain, 'How To JournalSpeak': thecureforchronicpain.com/journalspeak

Apps

- Curable: curablehealth.com/?gad=1&gclid=EAIaIQobChMI-_rB5PKM_wIVb4JLBR0wNQmsEAAYASAAEgJ02fD_BwE
- Nerva: try.nervaibs.com/hypnotherapy-nerva

Books

- *The Way Out: The Revolutionary, Scientifically Proven Approach to Heal Chronic Pain* by Alan Gordon
- *Endometriosis and Pelvic Pain* by Dr Susan Evans
- *Explain Pain Handbook: Protectometer* by David Butler and Lorimer Moseley (*Protectometer workbook* also available as iOS iPad App)

Podcasts

- One Thing Pain Podcast: shows.acast.com/one-thing-pain-podcast
- Tell Me About Your Pain: podcasts.apple.com/us/podcast/tell-me-about-your-pain/id1503847664
- Fempower Health: fempower-health.com/podcast/episode/2ca3daef/chronic-pelvic-pain-is-it-endometriosis-or-dr-peta-wright-and-dr-thea-bowler

Resources for understanding the mind–body connection and coming back to safety

Websites

- Deb Dana's Rhythm of Regulation (polyvagal theory): rhythmofregulation.com
- Jessica Maguire's 'Learn to repair your nervous system': jessicamaguire.com

Books

- *The Body Keeps the Score* by Bessel van der Kolk
- *My Grandmother's Hands* by Resmaa Menakem
- *The Polyvagal Theory in Therapy* by Deb Dana
- *Anchored* by Deb Dana
- *When the Body Says No* by Gabor Maté
- *The Myth of Normal* by Gabor Maté with Daniel Maté

Podcasts

- Ten Percent Happier: tenpercent.com/podcast-episode/ deb-dana-424
- The Jessica Golden Podcast: podcasts.apple.com/us/podcast/ 5-jessica-maguire-chronic-stress-trauma-the-nervous-system/ id1591927078?i=1000542611111 -
- We Can Do Hard Things: open.spotify.com/episode/ 6lqH0TEPyfpT9GPxcXEEMj

Body and cycle positive resources

Books

- *Bright Girl Guide: Use Your Period to Your Advantage* by Demi Spaccavento
- *Period Queen* by Lucy Peach
- *Women who Run with the Wolves* by Clarissa Pinkola Estés
- *Pussy, A Reclamation* by Regena Thomashauer
- *Cassandra Speaks* by Elizabeth Lesser

- *How to be a Woman* and *More than a Woman* by Caitlin Moran
- *Permission* by Lauren White
- *Untamed* by Glennon Doyle
- *The Period Repair Manual* and *The Hormone Repair Manual* by Lara Briden
- *The Fifth Vital Sign* by Lisa Hendrickson-Jack
- *In the Flo* by Alisa Vitti
- *Come as You Are* by Emily Nagowski
- *Burnout* by Emily and Amelia Nagowski

Other resources

Diet
- Tree of Life Nutrition: treeoflifenutrition.com.au/cookbook

Sleeping
- SA Health Insomnia Management Kit: sahealth.sa.gov.au/wps/wcm/connect/public+content/sa+health+internet/services/mental+health+and+drug+and+alcohol+services/drug+and+alcohol+services/for+health+professionals+dassa/sleep+problems+-+insomnia+management+kit

Mindfulness
- Future Learn: futurelearn.com/courses/mindfulness-wellbeing-performance
- Smiling Mind: smilingmind.com.au

Glossary

Ablative surgery – laparoscopic surgery that burns or lasers off a superficial endometriosis lesion.

Adenomyosis – the finding of cells similar to the lining of the uterus growing within the muscle layer of the wall of the uterus.

Allodynia – the perception of pain sensation from a non-painful stimulus.

Amitriptyline – a neuromodulating drug that reduces pain system hyper-sensitivity.

Anti-inflammatory diet – a diet rich in nutrients, fibre and phytochemicals to help reduce oxidative stress and inflammation in the body.

Autoimmune disease – describes conditions in which the body's immune system targets its own tissues.

Autonomic nervous system – the part of the nervous system that controls bodily function, not consciously directed, such as breathing, the heartbeat and digestion.

Bottom-up processing – the messages our brain gets from our body.

Central nervous system – includes the nerves that make up the brain and spinal cord.

Chronic pelvic pain – pain that persists on most days for greater than 3 months.

Cognitive behavioural therapy (CBT) – a common psychotherapy that links how you think and act with how you feel.

Complex PTSD – describes the dysregulation of the nervous system that occurs after repeated or ongoing traumas – often developmental traumas.

Corpus luteum – the name for the old follicle after release of the egg.

Curcumin – the active ingredient in the turmeric root that acts as an anti-inflammatory and can also block TLR4.

Dorsal vagal state – the back branch of the vagus nerve and another part of the parasympathetic nervous system. This is your freeze or shutdown state.

Dysbiosis – an imbalance in the make-up of the microbiome.

Dysregulated nervous system – describes being stuck in a survival nervous system state like fight/flight or freeze when there is no danger.

Dysmenorrhea – painful periods.

Embodiment – the connection between self and body.

Endometriosis – cells similar to the lining of the uterus that grow outside the uterus.

Excisional surgery – laparoscopic surgery that aims to surgically remove an endometriosis lesion in its entirety. This is imperative for deep endometriosis.

Eye movement desensitisation and reprocessing (EMDR) – a mental health technique involving moving your eyes in a specific way while you process traumatic memories.

Fight/flight – describes the mobilisation of the sympathetic nervous state.

Freeze – describes the immobilisation of the dorsal vagal state.

FODMAP – Fermentable, Oligo-, Di-, Mono-saccharides and Polyols are types of carbohydrates found in many foods.

Follicle Stimulating Hormone (FSH) – pituitary hormone that stimulates the growth of ovarian follicles.

Glial cells – non-neuron cells that help support, connect and protect the brain and nervous system.

GnRH (Gonadotropin-releasing hormone) agonists – block the messages from the brain to the ovaries to induce a temporary menopausal state. Zoladex, a monthly injection, is an example.

GnRH (Gonadotropin-releasing hormone) antagonists – block the messages from the brain to the ovaries to induce a temporary menopausal state. Ryeqo, a daily tablet, is an example – although this also contains add-back oestrogen and progestin.

Homeostasis – a physiological state of equilibrium and balance.

Hormonal IUD – an intrauterine device that contains a synthetic progestin.

Hyperalgesia – the perception of an amplified pain sensation.

Hypothalamic pituitary adrenal axis (HPA axis) – the communication system between the hypothalamus and the pituitary glands in the brain and the adrenal glands to produce stress hormones that activate a fight/flight response.

Hypothalamic pituitary ovarian axis (HPO axis) – the communication system between the hypothalamus and pituitary glands in the brain and the ovary, which controls ovulation.

Inflammation – the process by which the body recognises and removes harmful stimuli and begins the healing process. Can be acute or chronic. Chronic inflammation can lead to poor health outcomes.

Intestinal permeability – a condition where the lining of the gut becomes leaky, allowing parts of bacteria and toxins through where they can interact with the immune system.

Laparoscopy – keyhole surgery which uses a small camera to look and operate inside the pelvis.

Lipopolysaccharide (LPS) – part of the cell wall of E. coli bacteria that can induce changes in the immune system.

Low dose naltrexone – a drug that blocks opiate receptors in the brain and reduces neuroinflammation. It blocks TLR4 and increases the body's production of natural opiate.

Luteinising Hormone (LH) – pituitary hormone that causes ovulation.

Magnetic Resonance Imaging (MRI) – an imaging test that uses strong magnetic fields to take detailed images of the pelvis (or any part of the body). It is non-invasive and suitable for women who are not sexually active.

Microbiome – collection of microorganisms in a particular part of the body.

Monophasic – having a single phase.

Multidisciplinary team care – a model of care that comprises of a client and multiple health practitioners from different areas of health that communicate and collaborate to get the best care for their client.

NAC (N-Acetyl Cysteine) – a precursor to a powerful anti-oxidant called glutathione, which can reduce inflammation in the body.

Neurofeedback – a form of biofeedback which helps people to become consciously aware of, and change, their brain function. It can be helpful to rewire the effects of trauma on the brain.

Neuropathic pain – pain due to nerve damage.

Neuroplastic pain/pain system hypersensitivity – pain generated by the brain and nervous system.

Nociceptive pain – pain due to stimulation from trauma, inflammation and tissue damage.

Nociceptors – nerve cells that send 'possible threat' messages to the brain from real or perceived tissue damage.

Oestrogen – a hormone made by the ovarian follicles.

Opiates – strong painkillers like codeine, panadeine forte, endone, morphine and oxycodeine.

Oral contraceptive pill (OCP) – progestin and oestrogen containing birth control pill.

Ovarian follicle – the sac that contains an egg in the ovary.

Pain reprocessing therapy – an evidence-based approach to treat chronic pain that aims to rewire neural pathways in the brain in order to deactivate pain.

Palmitic acid – saturated fatty acid in meat, dairy, coconut and palm oil.

Parasympathetic nervous system – the rest and digest nervous system.

Pelvic floor overactivity/dysfunction – tense tight muscles around the vagina and anus.

Peripheral nerves – nerves outside the brain and spinal cord.

Polyvagal theory – describes the breakdown of the autonomic nervous system into 3 parts that relate to social behaviour and connection.

Post-traumatic stress disorder (PTSD) – describes the way a significant trauma lives on in the body causing nervous system dysregulation and preventing a person from being fully alive in the present.

Prebiotic – high-fibre foods that help to promote a healthy microbiome.

Predictive coding – a theory of brain function which tells us that the brain is constantly generating a mental model of the environment so, 'what we expect to experience we do experience.'

Probiotic – supplements containing beneficial good bacteria to improve gut health.

Progesterone – a hormone made by the ovary after ovulation.

Progestin – a synthetic version of progesterone, different types of progestins include Medroxyprogesterone acetate (MPA) – a synthetic progestin that suppresses the lining of the uterus, commonly sold as Depo-Provera, Mirena, Kyleena; the oral contraceptive pill (OCP) and Implanon contain MPA.

Prostaglandins – inflammatory chemicals released with periods and ovulation.

Retrograde menstruation – the process of menstrual blood flowing back into the pelvis at the time of a period.

Somatic pain – pain sensations coming from muscles, connective tissue, skin and bone.

Somatic therapy – a therapeutic approach that places importance on what we experience in the mind and the body as well as the connection between the two.

Somatic tracking – mindfulness and safety re-appraisal that helps people pay attention to painful sensations through a lens of safety which helps to deactivate the pain signal.

Sympathetic nervous system state – describes the hypothalamic-pituitary-adrenal axis and the fight or flight state.

TLR4 (toll-like receptor) – a cell that bridges the immune and nervous systems, increasing inflammation in the brain and dialling up pain pathways.

Top-down processing – how our brains interpret a situation based on knowledge, past experience and fear of the future.

Trans fat – a type of fat made by hydrogenation or processing of vegetable oils and can have an inflammatory effect in the body.

Transvaginal ultrasound (TV scan) – an ultrasound that uses a vaginal wand to take close-up pictures of the uterus and ovaries. Most women need to be sexually active to have a TV scan.

Trauma – the response to a deeply distressing or disturbing event that over-whelms a person's ability to cope, which causes feelings of helplessness, diminishes their sense of self and ability to feel fully alive in the present.

Ultrasound – a pelvic ultrasound is an imaging study to examine your ovaries and uterus. It uses sound waves and is safe and painless.

Vagus nerve – the large nerve on each side of the body that makes up the parasympathetic nervous system to influence heart rate, breathing, digestion, immune system and mood.

Ventral vagal state – the front branch of the vagus nerve and one part of the parasympathetic nervous system. This is your safe state.

Visceral pain – pain sensations coming from internal organs like the bladder, bowel, uterus or ovaries.

References

Introduction

P xiii   Pelvic pain affects one in five women . . .: SD Mathias et al., 'Chronic pelvic pain: prevalence, health-related quality of life, and economic correlates', *Obstetrics & gynecology*, vol. 87, no. 3, 1996, pp. 321–7.

Part 1: What causes pelvic pain?

P 6   Mild pain or discomfort in the . . .: M Armour et al., 'The prevalence and educational impact of pelvic and menstrual pain in Australia: A national online survey of 4202 young women aged 13–25 years', *Journal of pediatric and adolescent gynecology*, vol. 33, no. 5, 2020, pp. 511–8.

P 19   Worldwide, 14–32 per cent of women experience . . .: IJ Rowlands et al., 'Prevalence and incidence of endometriosis in Australian women: a data linkage cohort study', *BJOG: An international journal of obstetrics & gynaecology*, vol. 128, no. 4, 2021, pp. 657–65.

P 19   A recent Australian study of teenagers and . . .: A Randhawa et al., 'Secondary school girls' experiences of menstruation and awareness of endometriosis: a cross-sectional study', *Journal of pediatric and adolescent gynecology*, vol. 34, no. 5, 2021, pp. 643–8.

P 21   Women were seen as deformed or mutilated males . . .: C Nezhat et al., 'Endometriosis: ancient disease, ancient treatments', *Fertility and sterility*, vol. 98, no. 1, 2021, pp. S1–62.

P 22   A German doctor, Daniel Schrön, was perhaps the first . . .: ibid.

P 25   While estimates vary, most historical records indicate that around 50,000 women . . .: Julian Goodare, *The European witch-hunt*, Routledge, London, 2016.

P 30   But if, here in Australia at least, there is a push . . .: M Armour et al., 'Menstrual health literacy and management strategies in young women in Australia: a national online survey of young women aged 13–25 years', *Journal of pediatric and adolescent gynecology*, vol. 34, no. 2, 2021, pp. 135–43.

P 31   And around half of women who have a laparoscopy . . .: The Royal College of Obstetricians and Gynaecologists, *The initial management of chronic pelvic pain*, 2012, www.rcog.org.uk/media/muab2gj2/gtg_41.pdf.

P 31   In superficial endometriosis, the most common type . . .: AW Horne et al., 'Surgical removal of superficial peritoneal endometriosis for managing women with chronic pelvic pain: time for a rethink?', *BJOG: an international journal of obstetrics and gynaecology*, vol. 126, no. 12, 2019.

P 31   Of women diagnosed with endometriosis, 15 per cent . . .: ibid.

P 32   We know that this happens in almost 90 per cent . . .: J Halme et al., 'Retrograde menstruation in healthy women and in patients with endometriosis', *Obstetrics & gynecology*, vol. 64, no. 2, 1984, pp. 151–4.

P 34   The only positive predictive risk factor for endometriosis . . .: I Conroy et al., 'Pelvic pain: What are the symptoms and predictors for surgery, endometriosis and endometriosis severity', *Australian and New Zealand journal of obstetrics and gynaecology*, vol. 61, no. 5, 2021, pp. 765–72.

P 34   They activate the cells to produce pro–inflammatory chemicals . . .: KN Khan et al., 'Toll-like receptor system and endometriosis', *Journal of obstetrics and gynaecology research*, vol. 39, no. 8, 2013, pp. 1281–1292.; Y Azuma et al., 'Lipopolysaccharide promotes the development of murine endometriosis-like lesions via the nuclear factor-kappa B pathway', *American journal of reproductive immunology*, vol. 77, no. 4, 2017.

P 34   We know that the same molecular and cellular processes . . .: MJ Lacagnina et al., 'Toll-like receptors and their role in persistent pain', *Pharmacology & therapeutics*, vol. 184, 2018, pp. 145–58.

P 35   The first is through bacteria in the vagina . . .: KN Khan et al., 'Bacterial contamination hypothesis: a new concept in endometriosis', *Reproductive medicine and biology*, vol. 17, no. 2, 2018, pp. 125–33.

P 35   Research has shown that women with endometriosis often have lower levels . . .: B Ata et al., 'The endobiota study: comparison of vaginal, cervical and gut microbiota between women with stage 3/4 endometriosis and healthy controls', *Scientific reports*, vol. 9, no. 1, 2019.

P 36   If the integrity of the intestinal wall is disturbed . . .: D Viganó et al., 'How is small bowel permeability in endometriosis patients? A case control pilot study', *Gynecological endocrinology*, vol. 36, no. 11, 2020, pp. 1010–14.

P 36   These immune cells such as TLR4 can then migrate . . .: I Jiang et al., 'Intricate connections between the microbiota and endometriosis', *International journal of molecular sciences*, vol. 22, no. 11, 2021.

P 36   TLR4 cells also increase inflammation in the brain . . .: MJ Lacagnina et al., 'Toll-like receptors and their role in persistent pain', *Pharmacology & therapeutics*, vol. 184, 2018, pp. 145–58.

P 36   There is also recent evidence (albeit in mice), suggesting . . .: Muraoka, A. et al., 'Fusobacterium infection facilitates the development of endometriosis through the phenotypic transition of endometrial fibroblasts', *Science Translational Medicine*, vol. 15, no. 700, 2023, eadd1531.

P 37   This gut–immune system connection may also be implicated . . .: M Porpora et al., 'High prevalence of autoimmune diseases in women with endometriosis: a case-control study', *Gynecological endocrinology*, vol. 36, no. 4, 2020, pp. 356–59.

P 37   Women who have severe disease, with large endometriomas . . .: AW Horne et al., 'Surgical removal of superficial peritoneal endometriosis for managing women with chronic pelvic pain: time for a rethink?', *BJOG: an international journal of obstetrics and gynaecology*, vol. 126, no. 12, 2019.

P 37   Even so, there is little correlation between severity of disease . . .: I Conroy et al., 'Pelvic pain: What are the symptoms and predictors for surgery, endometriosis and endometriosis severity', *Australian and New Zealand Journal of obstetrics and gynaecology*, vol. 61, no. 5, 2021, pp. 765–72.

P 38   In fact, a study following up women who had no symptoms . . .: MH Moen and T Stokstad, 'A long-term follow-up study of women with asymptomatic endo-metriosis diagnosed incidentally at sterilization', *Fertility and sterility*, vol. 78, no. 4, 2002, pp. 773–6.

P 38   Some studies have reported the presence of endometriosis lesions . . .: J Rawson, 'Prevalence of endometriosis in asymptomatic women', *The Journal of reproductive medicine*, vol. 36, no. 7, 1991, pp. 513–5.

P 38   In one of these studies – conducted in the 90s – up to 44 per cent . . .: ibid.

P 40   A retrospective clinical study showed that in women with endometriomas . . .: KN Khan et al., 'Pelvic pain in women with ovarian endometrioma is mostly associated with coexisting peritoneal lesions', *Human reproduction*, vol. 28, no. 1, 2013, pp. 109–18.

P 41   While the conventional understanding is that laparoscopy is necessary to diagnose endometriosis . . .: M Leonardi et al., 'Transvaginal ultrasound can accurately predict the American society of reproductive medicine stage of endometriosis assigned at laparoscopy', *Journal of minimally invasive gynecology*, vol. 27, no. 7, 2020, pp. 1581–7.; T Indrielle-Kelly et al., 'Diagnostic accuracy of ultrasound and MRI in the mapping of deep pelvic endometriosis using the International Deep Endometriosis Analysis (IDEA) consensus', *BioMed research international*, vol. 2020, 2020.

P 41   A 2020 study looked at laparoscopy findings from 150 women . . .: N Tempest et al., 'Laparoscopic outcomes after normal clinical and ultrasound findings in young women with chronic pelvic pain: a cross-sectional study', *Journal of clinical medicine*, vol. 9, no. 8, 2020.

P 42   The authors concluded that 'women should be informed of the multifactorial nature of chronic pelvic pain ...' . . .: ibid.

P 42   An amalgamation of clinical trials where laparoscopies were performed . . .: JLH Hans Evers, 'Is adolescent endometriosis a progressive disease that needs to be diagnosed and treated?' *Human reproduction (Oxford, England)*, vol. 28, no. 8, 2013.

P 42   Another study did laparoscopies 3 months apart and found . . .: RF Harrison and C Barry-Kinsella, 'Efficacy of medroxyprogesterone treatment in infertile women with endometriosis: a prospective, randomized, placebo-controlled study', *Fertility and sterility*, vol. 74, no. 1, 2000, pp. 24–30.

P 43   Even deep endometriosis around the rectum and vagina . . .: P Vercellini et al., 'The effect of surgery for symptomatic endometriosis: the other side of the story', *Human reproduction update*, vol. 15, no. 2, 2009, pp. 177–88.

P 43   There is no evidence to support doing laparoscopic surgery prior to IVF . . .: AW Horne and SA Missmer, 'Pathophysiology, diagnosis, and management of endometriosis', *BMJ (clinical research ed.)*, vol. 379, 2022.

P 43   Current evidence suggests that pregnancy rates with IVF . . .: HA Homer, 'Effects of endometriosis on in vitro fertilisation: Myth or reality?', *Australian and New Zealand journal of obstetrics and gynaecology*, vol. 63, no. 1, 2023, pp. 3–5.

P 48   The rate of arterial thrombosis (a blood clot in an arteries) . . .: L Manzoli et al., 'Oral contraceptives and venous thromboembolism: a systematic review and meta-analysis', *Drug safety*, vol. 35, 2012, pp. 191–205.

P 48   This still only means, however, that roughly 185 women . . .: National Cancer Institute, *Oral contraceptives and cancer risk*, 2018, www.cancer.gov/about-cancer/causes-prevention/risk/hormones/oral-contraceptives-fact-sheet

P 49   Studies on the effect of the Pill . . .: CW Skovlund et al., 'Association of hormonal contraception with depression', *JAMA psychiatry*, vol. 73, no. 11, 2016, pp. 1154–62.

P 49   Research has also shown that starting the Pill . . .: C Anderl et al., 'Oral contraceptive use in adolescence predicts lasting vulnerability to depression in adulthood', *Journal of child psychology and psychiatry*, vol. 61, no. 2, 2020, pp. 148–56.

P 50   A recent Australian study also reported that women . . .: LC Arthur and KR Blake, 'Fertility predicts self-development-oriented competitiveness in naturally cycling women but not hormonal contraceptive users', *Adaptive human behavior and physiology*, 2022, pp. 1–31.

P 50   Some new research also suggests that women . . .: BJ Crespi and SF Evans, 'Prenatal origins of endometriosis pathology and pain: Reviewing the evidence of a role for low testosterone', *Journal of pain research*, vol. 16, 2023, pp. 307–16.

P 50   While a 2014 Cochrane review . . .: LM Lopez et al., 'Steroidal contraceptives: effect on bone fractures in women', *Cochrane database of systematic reviews 2014*, issue 6.

P 51   Unless they also make changes to their diet and lifestyle ...: E Diamanti-Kandarakis et al., 'A modern medical quandary: polycystic ovary syndrome, insulin resistance, and oral contraceptive pills', *The journal of clinical endocrinology & metabolism*, vol. 88, no. 5, 2003, pp. 1927–32.

P 54   They found that both the placebo and Provera ...: RF Harrison and C Barry-Kinsella, 'Efficacy of medroxyprogesterone treatment in infertile women with endometriosis: a prospective, randomized, placebo-controlled study', *Fertility and sterility*, vol. 74, no. 1, 2000, pp. 24–30.

P 56   Only one-tenth of the progestin dose can ...: AF Alavi and F Farnam, 'Weight changes 12–18 months after IUD and DMPA usage: A retrospective cohort study', *The Iranian Journal of Obstetrics, Gynecology and Infertility*, vol. 23, no. 7, 2020, pp. 39–46. 2020

P 56   Studies on the impact of Mirena on mood and ...: CW Skovlund et al., 'Association of hormonal contraception with depression', *JAMA psychiatry*, vol. 73, no. 11, 2016, pp. 1154–62.

P 56   A recent meta–analysis showed variable results ...: M Elsayed et al., 'The potential association between psychiatric symptoms and the use of levonorgestrel intrauterine devices (LNG-IUDs): A systematic review', *The world journal of biological psychiatry*, 2022, p. 1–19.

P 59   A meta-analysis on medical treatments and pelvic pain showed ...: CM Becker et al., 'Reevaluating response and failure of medical treatment of endometriosis: a systematic review', *Fertility and sterility*, vol. 108, no. 1, 2017, pp. 125–36.

P 62   The result was that the Pill became the first medication ...: M Williams-Deane and LS Potter, 'Current oral contraceptive use instructions: an analysis of patient package inserts', *Family Planning Perspectives*, vol. 24, no. 3, 1992, pp. 111–5.

P 62   Someone even suggested during the hearings ...: Mike Gaskins, *In the Name of the Pill*, America, Mike Gaskins, 2019.

P 63   Even a high-quality Cochrane review concluded ...: J Brown et al., 'Oral contraceptives for pain associated with endometriosis', *Cochrane database of systematic reviews 2018*, vol. 5, no. 5, 2018.

P 65   Up to half of women who have their lesions excised ...: P Vercellini et al., 'The effect of surgery for symptomatic endometriosis: the other side of the story', *Human reproduction update*, vol. 15, issue 2, 2009, pp. 177–88.

P 66   While an 80 per cent improvement in pain ...: J Abbott et al., 'Laparoscopic excision of endometriosis: a randomized, placebo-controlled trial', *Fertility and sterility*, vol. 82, no. 4, 2004, pp. 878–84.

P 66   They found that pain improved in 80 per cent of women ...: J Abbott et al., 'Laparoscopic excision of endometriosis: a randomized, placebo-controlled trial', *Fertility and sterility*, vol. 82, no. 4, 2004, pp 878–84.

P 67   This shows again that endometriosis is not always progressive ...: P Vercellini et al., 'The effect of surgery for symptomatic endometriosis: the other side of the story', *Human reproduction update*, vol. 15, issue 2, 2009, pp. 177–88.

P 67   A 2020 systematic Cochrane review of laparoscopic surgery ...: JMN Duffy et al., 'Laparoscopic surgery for endometriosis', *The cochrane database of systematic reviews*, vol. 4, 2014.

P 67   Studies tell us that women with cyclical symptoms ...: A Harris et al., 'Endometriosis-related pelvic pain following laparoscopic surgical treatment', *Journal of endometriosis and pelvic pain disorders*, vol. 12, no. 3–4, 2020, pp. 151–7.

P 68   On the other hand, women with chronic pelvic pain ...: ibid.

P 68   This is something worth remembering when we consider the ...: AW Horne et al., 'Surgical removal of superficial peritoneal endometriosis for managing women with chronic pelvic pain: time for a rethink?', *BJOG: an international journal of obstetrics and gynaecology*, vol. 126, no. 12, 2019.

P 68   A Cochrane review showed that the effect . . .: JMN Duffy et al., 'Laparoscopic surgery for endometriosis', *The cochrane database of systematic reviews*, 2014.

P 68   A 2000 letter to the editor of the *British Medical Journal* . . .: D Redwine et al., 'Evidence on endometriosis. Elitism about randomised controlled trials is inappropriate', *BMJ (Clinical research ed.)*, vol. 321, no. 7268, 2000, p. 1077–8.

P 73   Orthopaedics – a specialty that deals with bones . . .: A Louw et al. 'Sham surgery in orthopedics: a systematic review of the literature', *Pain medicine*, vol. 18, no. 4, 2017, pp. 736–50.

P 74   Other operations such as spinal fusion . . .: M Englund et al. 'Incidental meniscal findings on knee MRI in middle-aged and elderly persons', *New England journal of medicine*, vol. 359, no. 11, 2008, pp. 1108–15.

P 74   Just as with endometriosis, there is evidence . . .: MC Jensen et al., 'Magnetic resonance imaging of the lumbar spine in people without back pain', *New England journal of medicine*, vol. 331, no. 2, 1994, pp. 69–73.

P 74   So far there is little evidence that shows surgery . . .: J Jarrell et al., 'Laparoscopy and reported pain among patients with endometriosis.' *Journal of obstetrics and gynaecology Canada*, vol. 27, no. 5, 2005, pp. 477–85.; AW Horne et al., 'Surgical removal of superficial peritoneal endometriosis for managing women with chronic pelvic pain: time for a rethink?', *BJOG: an international journal of obstetrics and gynaecology*, vol. 126, no. 12, 2019.

P 74   One, occurring in Denmark, is designed as a double–blinded . . .: H Marschall et al., 'Is laparoscopic excision for superficial peritoneal endometriosis helpful or harmful? Protocol for a double-blinded, randomised, placebo-controlled, three-armed surgical trial', *BMJ open*, vol. 12, no. 11, 2022.

P 74   This particular trial is comparing levels of pelvic pain . . .: ibid

P 74   The other is a large multicentre trial . . .: AW Horne et al., 'Surgical removal of superficial peritoneal endometriosis for managing women with chronic pelvic pain: time for a rethink?', *BJOG: an international journal of obstetrics and gynaecology*, vol. 126, no. 12, 2019.

P 77   The recent Australian *Endometriosis Clinical Practice Guidelines* stated . . .: RANZCOG, *Australian clinical practice guideline for the diagnosis and management of endometriosis*, RANZCOG, Melbourne, 2021.

P 82   As far back as 1947, the World Health Organization's Constitution . . .: World Health Organization, 'Constitution of the World Health Organization', *Chronicle of the World Health Organization*, vol. 1, no. 1–2, 1947, p. 29.

P 82   In the 1990s, US doctor and holistic treatment advocate . . .: AR Tarlov, *Social determinants of health: The sociobiological translation*, Routledge, London, 2002, p. 72.

P 96   We know that pain is worse when a person is tired . . .: J Woelk et al., 'I'm tired and it hurts! Sleep quality and acute pain response in a chronic pain population', *Sleep medicine*, vol. 67, 2020, pp. 28–32.

P 96   One study showed that the somatosensory cortex . . .: E Kross et al., 'Social rejection shares somatosensory representations with physical pain', *Proceedings of the national academy of sciences*, vol. 108, no. 15, 2011, pp. 6270–5.

P 96   Researchers also measured a 60–90 per cent decrease . . .: AJ Krause et al., 'The pain of sleep loss: a brain characterization in humans', *Journal of Neuroscience*, vol. 39, no. 12, 2019, pp. 2291–300.

P 96   Sleep deprivation also increases production of cortisol . . .: KP Wright Jr et al., 'Influence of sleep deprivation and circadian misalignment on cortisol, inflammatory markers, and cytokine balance', *Brain, behavior, and immunity*, vol. 47, 2015, pp. 24–34.

P 97   In fact, in a recent study, almost 80 per cent . . .: A Ryan et al., 'Central sensitisation in pelvic pain: A cohort study', *Australian and New Zealand journal of obstetrics and gynaecology*, vol. 62, no. 6, 2022, pp. 868–74.

P 98   Normal sensitisation and Pain system hypersensitivity (images): CJ Woolf, 'Central sensitization: implications for the diagnosis and treatment of pain', *Pain*, vol. 152, supplement, 2011, pp. S2–S15.

P 98   People whose acute pain becomes chronic pain . . .: CY Casey et al., 'Transition from acute to chronic pain and disability: a model including cognitive, affective, and trauma factors', *Pain*, vol. 134, no. 1–2, 2008, pp. 69–79.; S Kempke et al., 'Self-critical perfectionism and its relationship to fatigue and pain in the daily flow of life in patients with chronic fatigue syndrome', *Psychological medicine*, vol. 43, no. 5, 2013, pp. 995–1002.

P 101   Neuroplasticity means that while chronic pain can be learned . . .: A Mansour et al., 'Chronic pain: the role of learning and brain plasticity', *Restorative neurology and neuroscience*, vol. 32, no. 1, 2014, pp. 129–39.

P 108   There is evidence that the language we use . . .: D Wilson et al., 'Language and the pain experience', *Physiotherapy research international*, vol. 14, no. 1, 2009, pp. 56–65.

p 112   In my view, polyvagal theory, proposed in the mid-1990s . . .: Stephen W Porges, *The pocket guide to the polyvagal theory: The transformative power of feeling safe*, W. W. Norton & Company, Inc., New York, NY, 2017.

P 116   This not only causes more digestive symptoms . . .: SR Dube et al., 'Cumulative childhood stress and autoimmune diseases in adults', *Psychosomatic medicine*, vol. 71, no. 2, 2009, p. 243.

P 116   In fact, a recent study on rats showed . . .: Q Long et al., 'Chronic stress accelerates the development of endometriosis in mouse through adrenergic receptor B2', *Human reproduction*, vol. 31, no. 11, 2016, pp. 2506–19.

P 129   The Adverse Childhood Experiences (ACE) study . . .: VJ Felitti et al., 'Relationship of childhood abuse and household dysfunction to many of the leading causes of death in adults: The Adverse Childhood Experiences (ACE) study', *American journal of preventive medicine*, vol. 14, no. 4, 1998, pp. 245–58.

P 129   She said, 'Overweight is to be overlooked . . . '. . .: VJ Felitti, 'Origins of the ACE study', *American journal of preventive medicine*, vol. 56, no. 6, 2019, pp. 787–9.

P 130   It might sound obvious that being poorly treated . . .: VJ Felitti et al., 'Relationship of childhood abuse and household dysfunction to many of the leading causes of death in adults: The Adverse Childhood Experiences (ACE) Study', *American journal of preventive medicine*, vol. 14, no. 4, 1998, pp. 245–58.

P 130   Later studies have shown that early life trauma . . .: CT Tay et al., 'Psychiatric comorbidities and adverse childhood experiences in women with self-reported polycystic ovary syndrome: an Australian population-based study', *Psychoneuroendocrinology*, vol. 116, 2020.; A Danese and SJ Lewis, 'Psychoneuroimmunology of early-life stress: the hidden wounds of childhood trauma?', *Neuropsychopharmacology*, vol. 42, no. 1, 2017, pp. 99–114.

P 131   The types of exposures more likely to predispose people . . .: CDC, Kaiser Permanente & ACE study (unpublished survey data), US Department of Health and Human Services & Centers for Disease Control, Atlanta, Georgia, 2016; B C Groenewald et al., 'Adverse childhood experiences and chronic pain among children and adolescents in the United States', *PAIN Reports*, vol. 5, no. 5, p. e839, 2020; S M Nelson et al., 'A Conceptual Framework for Understanding the Role of Adverse Childhood Experiences in Pediatric Chronic Pain', *The Clinical Journal of Pain,* vol. 33 no. 3, pp, 264–270, 2017.

P 131   A multitude of studies has found an increased likelihood . . .: C Heim et al., 'Abuse-related post-traumatic stress disorder and alterations of the hypothalamic-pituitary-adrenal axis in women with chronic pelvic pain', *Psychosomatic medicine*, vol. 60, no. 3, 1998, pp. 309–18.; D Moussaoui et al., 'Short review on adverse childhood experiences, pelvic pain and endometriosis', *Journal of gynecology obstetrics and human reproduction*, vol. 52, no. 6, 2023.; M Bourdon et al.,

'Severe pelvic pain is associated with sexual abuse experienced during childhood and/or adolescence irrespective of the presence of endometriosis', *Human reproduction (Oxford, England)*, dead119, 2023.; D Moussaoui and SR Grover, 'The association between childhood adversity and risk of dysmenorrhoea, pelvic pain and dyspareunia in adolescents and young adults: a systematic review', *Journal of pediatric and adolescent gynecology*, vol. 35, no. 5, 2022, pp. 567–74.

P 131 A 2018 study even found that women . . .: HR Harris et al., 'Early life abuse and risk of endometriosis', *Human reproduction*, vol. 33, no. 9, 2018, pp. 1657–68.

P 132 More than 18 per cent of children with more . . .: CB Groenewald et al., 'Adverse childhood experiences and chronic pain among children and adolescents in the United States', *Pain reports*, vol. 5, no. 5, 2020.

P 132 A 2022 systematic review concluded that there . . .: D Moussaoui and SR Grover, 'The association between childhood adversity and risk of dysmenorrhoea, pelvic pain and dyspareunia in adolescents and young adults: a systematic review', *Journal of pediatric and adolescent gynecology*, vol. 35, no. 5, 2022, pp. 567–74.

P 132 The same group published a paper in 2023 . . .: D Moussaoui et al., 'Short review on adverse childhood experiences, pelvic pain and endometriosis', *Journal of gynecology obstetrics and human reproduction*, vol. 52, no. 6, 2023.

P 133 This theory was borne out in a 2023 study . . .: M Bourdon et al., 'Severe pelvic pain is associated with sexual abuse experienced during childhood and/or adolescence irrespective of the presence of endometriosis', *Human reproduction (Oxford, England)*, dead119, 2023.

P 133 Generally, most studies have found that girls . . .: MT Baglivio et al., 'The prevalence of Adverse Childhood Experiences (ACE) in the lives of juvenile offenders', *Journal of juvenile justice*, vol. 3, no. 2, 2014.

P 134 He says that, 'Early childhood mechanisms of self-suppression . . . '...: Gabor Maté with Daniel Maté, *The myth of normal: Trauma, illness & healing in a toxic culture*, Random House, London, 2022.

P 135 This is auto-immune disease and it is well-known . . .: SR Dube et al., 'Cumulative childhood stress and autoimmune diseases in adults', *Psychosomatic medicine*, vol. 71, no. 2, 2009.

P 136 A recent study looking at the impacts of early life stress . . .: S Salberg et al., 'Pain in the developing brain: early life factors alter nociception and neurobiological function in adolescent rats', *Cerebral cortex communications*, vol. 2, issue 2, 2021.

P 136 Previous work on adolescent pain conditions showed . . .: CH Dennis et al., 'Adverse childhood experiences in mothers with chronic pain and intergenerational impact on children', *Journal of pain*, vol. 20, 2019, pp. 1209–17.

P 136 Other human studies have also demonstrated that exposure . . .: A Saleh et al., 'Effects of early life stress on depression, cognitive performance and brain morphology', *Psychological medicine*, vol. 47, no. 1, 2017, pp. 171–81.

P 136   Mirroring the rat study, a plethora of evidence shows . . .: PH Croll, et al., 'Better diet quality relates to larger brain tissue volumes: the Rotterdam study', *Neurology*, vol. 90, no. 24, 2018.

P 137 There is lots of research now that the resultant inflammation . . .: MJ Lacagnina et al., 'Toll-like receptors and their role in persistent pain', *Pharmacology & therapeutics*, vol. 184, 2018, pp. 145–58.

P 137 There is scientific evidence that stress eating is real.: YH Yau and MN Potenza, 'Stress and eating behaviors', *Minerva endocrinologica*, vol. 38, no. 3, 2013.

P 140 Women who start the Pill in adolescence . . .: J Gervasio et al., 'The effect of oral contraceptive use on cortisol reactivity to the Trier Social Stress Test: A meta-analysis', *Psychoneuroendocrinology*, vol. 136, 2022.

P 140 In addition, while there is evidence that fluctuating oestrogen . . .: S Bazin et al., 'Vulvar vestibulitis syndrome: an exploratory case-control study', *Obstetrics & gynecology*, vol. 83, no. 1, 1994, pp. 47–50.

P 140   There is even emerging evidence that low testosterone states . . .: BJ Crespi and SF Evans, 'Prenatal origins of endometriosis pathology and pain: reviewing the evidence of a role for low testosterone', *Journal of pain research*, 2023, pp. 307–16.

P 140   A recent report showed that more than 38 per cent . . .: National Institute of Mental Health, *Mental health information: any anxiety disorder*, accessed June 2023, nimh.nih.gov

P 142   As one doctor has written on the effects of childhood trauma . . .: WC Jackson, 'Connecting the dots: how adverse childhood experiences predispose to chronic pain', *Practical pain management*, vol. 20, no. 3, 2020.

Part 2: A practical pathway to true healing

P 149   Numerous studies have shown these to be as effective as ibuprofen . . .: G Ozgoli et al., 'Comparison of effects of ginger, mefenamic acid, and ibuprofen on pain in women with primary dysmenorrhea', *Journal of alternative and complementary medicine*, vol. 15, no. 2, 2009, pp. 129–32.

P 150   This combination has been found to be as effective at reducing pain . . .: G Ozgoli et al., 'Comparison of effects of ginger, mefenamic acid, and ibuprofen on pain in women with primary dysmenorrhea', *The journal of alternative and complementary medicine*, vol. 15, no. 2, 2009, pp. 129–132.; S Rahman et al., 'Efficacy of oral Tranexamic Acid versus combined oral contraceptives for heavy menstrual bleeding', *Cureus*, vol. 13, no. 10, 2021.

P 150   There is no one-size-fits-all endometriosis diet but . . .: R Estruch, 'Anti-inflammatory effects of the Mediterranean diet: the experience of the PREDIMED study', *Proceedings of the nutrition society*, vol. 69, no. 3, 2010, pp. 333–40.; F Sofi et al., 'Adherence to Mediterranean diet and health status: meta-analysis.' *BMJ (Clinical research ed.)*, vol. 337, 2008.; G Merra et al., 'Influence of Mediterranean diet on human gut microbiota.' *Nutrients*, vol. 13, no. 1, 2020.

P 154   Foods containing wheat or gluten may impair . . .: DS Mills, 'A conundrum: wheat and gluten avoidance and its implication with endometriosis patients.' *Fertility and sterility*, vol. 96, no. 3, 2011.

P 154   Dairy: While many studies actually suggest that high dairy . . .: K Nirgianakis et al., 'Effectiveness of dietary interventions in the treatment of endometriosis: a systematic review', *Reproductive sciences*, vol, 29, no. 1, 2022.

P 154   Pesticides and other chemicals in food . . .: K Upson et al., 'Organochlorine pesticides and risk of endometriosis: findings from a population-based case-control study', *Environmental health perspectives*, vol. 121, no. 11–12, 2013, pp. 1319–24.

P 155   The latest research on IBS tells us . . .: DH Vasant and PJ Whorwell, 'Gut-focused hypnotherapy for functional gastrointestinal disorders: Evidence-base, practical aspects, and the Manchester protocol', *Neurogastroenterology & motility*, vol. 31, no. 8, 2019.

P 156   Curcumin (turmeric), which in endometriosis lesions accelerates . . .: A Vallée and Y Lecarpentier, 'Curcumin and endometriosis', *International journal of molecular sciences*, vol. 21, no. 7, 2020.; M Boozari et al., 'Impact of curcumin on toll-like receptors', *Journal of cellular physiology*, vol. 234, no. 8, 2019.

P 156   Zinc, which repairs intestinal permeability to help . . .: Y Shao et al., 'Zinc enhances intestinal epithelial barrier function through the PI3K/AKT/mTOR signaling pathway in Caco-2 cells', *Journal of nutritional biochemistry*', vol. 43, 2017, pp. 18–26.

P 156   The usual dose is 30 milligrams a day taken with food.: MSG Naz et al., 'The effect of micronutrients on pain management of primary dysmenorrhea: a systematic review and meta-analysis', *Journal of caring sciences*, vol. 9, no. 1, 2020.

P 156   magnesium, taken daily or with periods . . .: H-J Shin et al., 'Magnesium and pain', *Nutrients*, vol. 12, no. 8, 2020.

P 156 In a very small 2013 study of 92 women . . .: MG Porpora et al., 'A promise in the treatment of endometriosis: an observational cohort study on ovarian endometrioma reduction by N-acetylcysteine', *Evidence-based complementary and alternative medicine*, vol. 2013, article no. 240702, 2013.

P 156 I usually recommend magnesium glycinate because . . .: Lara Briden, *8 ways magnesium rescues hormones*, 30 Mar 2014, www.larabriden.com/8-ways-that-magnesium-rescues-hormones

P 156 fish oil (omega–3), which reduces prostaglandin . . .: B Deutch et al., 'Menstrual discomfort in Danish women reduced by dietary supplements of omega-3 PUFA and B12 (fish oil or seal oil capsules)', *Nutrition research*, vol. 20, no. 5, 2000, pp. 621–31.

P 156 vitamin D; several studies have shown . . .: F Abdi et al., 'Role of vitamin D and calcium in the relief of primary dysmenorrhea: a systematic review', *Obstetrics & gynecology science*, vol. 64, no. 1, 2021, pp. 13–26.

P 156 probiotics, which are helpful in restoring. . .: S Khodaverdi et al., 'Beneficial effects of oral lactobacillus on pain severity in women suffering from endometriosis: A pilot placebo-controlled randomized clinical trial.' *International journal of fertility & sterility*, vol. 13, no. 3, 2019.

P 158 It's also known to decrease cortisol and insulin . . .: JM Mullington et al., 'Sleep loss and inflammation', *Best practice & research clinical endocrinology & metabolism*, vol. 24, no. 5, 2010, pp. 775–84.

P 158 Chemicals such as phthalates, dioxins and PCBs . . .: X Wen et al., 'The risk of endometriosis after exposure to endocrine-disrupting chemicals: a meta-analysis of 30 epidemiology studies', *Gynecological endocrinology*, vol. 35, no. 8, 2019, pp. 645–50.

P 161 A recent survey of gynaecologists in the UK . . .: HW Leow et al., '45% of UK gynaecologists think chronic pelvic pain is managed badly', *European journal of obstetrics and gynecology and reproductive biology*, vol. 224, 2018, pp. 200–202.; J Price et al., 'Attitudes of women with chronic pelvic pain to the gynaecological consultation: a qualitative study', *BJOG: An international journal of obstetrics & gynaecology*, vol. 113, no. 4, 2006, pp. 446–52.

P 161 In women diagnosed with endometriosis . . .: P Vercellini et al., 'The effect of surgery for symptomatic endometriosis: the other side of the story', *Human reproduction update*, vol. 15, no. 2, 2009, pp. 177–88.

P 172 The available evidence shows it can have significant effects . . .: J Abbott, 'Gynecological indications for the use of botulinum toxin in women with chronic pelvic pain', *Toxicon*, vol. 54, no. 5, 2009, pp. 647–53.

P 180 A chronically dysregulated nervous system is . . .: R Tian et al., 'A possible change process of inflammatory cytokines in the prolonged chronic stress and its ultimate implications for health', *The scientific world journal*, vol. 2014, 2014.

P 187 Journaling is an evidence-based practice that can . . .: M Sohal et al., 'Efficacy of journaling in the management of mental illness: a systematic review and meta-analysis', *Family medicine and community health*, vol. 10, no. 1, 2022.

P 187 Even if no one sees it but you . . .: ibid.

P 187 Nicole Sachs is a psychotherapist and writer whose technique . . .: The Cure for Chronic Pain, *Nicole Sachs, LCSW*, accessed June 2023, thecureforchronicpain.com/aboutnicole

P 187 Nicole writes that 'once emotions are given . . .' . . .: ibid.

P 188 Although this is intuitive, music therapy . . .: S Aalbers et al., 'Music therapy for depression', *Cochrane database of systematic reviews*, issue 11, 2017.

P 188 There is even research showing that humming . . .: G Trivedi et al., 'Humming (simple bhramari pranayama) as a stress buster: A holter-based study to analyze heart rate variability (HRV) parameters during bhramari, physical activity, emotional stress, and sleep', *Cureus*, vol. 15, no. 4, 2023.

P 195   Bruce Perry, a psychiatrist and one of the world's leading expert . . .: Dr Bruce Perry and Oprah Winfrey, *What Happened to you?: Conversations on trauma, resilience and healing*, Bluebird, London, 2021.

P 196   'The parent-child connection is the most powerful . . .': Bessel van der Kolk, *Psychological trauma*, American Psychiatric Press, Inc., Washington, DC, 2003.

P 202   Renowned trauma expert, Bessel van der Kolk, recommends . . .: M Kuhfuß et al., 'Somatic experiencing – effectiveness and key factors of a body-oriented trauma therapy: a scoping literature review', *European journal of psychotraumatology*, vol. 12, no. 1, 2021.; Bessel van der Kolk, *The body keeps the score*, Viking, New York, NY, 2014.

P 207   Lots of research shows that chronic pain improves . . .: A Meulders 'Fear in the context of pain: Lessons learned from 100 years of fear conditioning research', *Behaviour research and therapy*, vol. 131, 2020.

P 207   Modern pain science tells us that pain education . . .: GL Moseley and DS Butler, 'Fifteen years of explaining pain: the past, present, and future', *The journal of pain*, vol. 16, no. 9, 2015, pp. 807–13.

P 207   We also know that people who understand . . .: PJ Köppen et al., 'Health literacy, pain intensity and pain perception in patients with chronic pain', *Wiener Klinische Wochenschrift*, vol. 130, 2018, pp. 23–30.

P 210   A 2022 clinical trial on patients with back pain . . .: YK Ashar et al., 'Effect of pain reprocessing therapy vs placebo and usual care for patients with chronic back pain: a randomized clinical trial', *JAMA psychiatry*, vol. 79, no. 1, 2022, pp. 13–23.

P 211   'Predictive sensory processing can take expectations of pain and make pain.': Suzanne O'Sullivan, *The sleeping beauties: And other stories of mystery illness*, Picador, London, 2021.

P 211   A recent New Zealand study showed that . . .: A Ryan et al., 'Central sensitisation in pelvic pain: A cohort study', *Australian and New Zealand journal of obstetrics and gynaecology*, vol. 62, no. 6, 2022, pp. 868–74.

P 211   Once we accept that chronic pelvic pain . . .: Howard Schubiner and Michael Betzold, *Unlearn your pain*, Mind Body Publishing, Pleasant Ridge, MI, 2010.

P 216   Bessel van der Kolk showed in his research that yoga . . .: Bessel van der Kolk, *The body keeps the score*, Viking, New York, NY, 2014.

P 216   Yoga for patients with chronic pelvic pain . . .: AV Gonçalves et al., 'The practice of hatha yoga for the treatment of pain associated with endometriosis', *The journal of alternative and complementary medicine*, vol. 23, no. 1, 2017, pp. 45–52.

P 216   Yoga practice has been shown to increase levels . . .: S Varambally et al., 'Yoga for psychiatric disorders: from fad to evidence-based intervention?' *The British journal of psychiatry*, vol. 216, no. 6, 2020, pp. 291–93.

P 216   Studies have also shown improvements in chronic pain . . .: B Hickman et al., 'Dance for chronic pain conditions: A systematic review', *Pain medicine*, vol. 23, no. 12, 2022, pp. 2022–41.

P 217   Writing about somatic experiencing, psychologist Peter Levine . . .: Peter A. Levine, *Waking the tiger: Healing trauma*, North Atlantic Books, Berkeley, CA, 1997.

P 223   A few studies have shown some benefit . . .: CC Bittelbrunn et al., 'Pelvic floor physical therapy and mindfulness: approaches for chronic pelvic pain in women – a systematic review and meta-analysis', *Archives of gynecology and obstetrics*, vol. 307, no. 3, 2023, pp. 663–72.

P 224   Having said that, a recent 2022 systematic review showed . . .: DA van Reijn-Baggen et al., 'Pelvic floor physical therapy for pelvic floor hypertonicity: a systematic review of treatment efficacy', *Sexual medicine reviews*, vol. 10, no. 2, 2022, pp. 209–30.

Part 3: Transcendence

P 243   The evidence that pelvic pain is best managed . . .: R Wilkinson et al., 'Impact of a persistent pelvic pain clinic: emergency attendances following multidisciplinary management of persistent pelvic pain', *Australian and New Zealand journal of obstetrics and gynaecology*, vol. 61, no. 4, 2021, pp. 612–15.

P 254   Cultural anthropologist, Alma Gottlieb, in her essay 'Menstrual Taboos' . . .: A Gottlieb, 'Menstrual taboos: Moving beyond the curse', *The Palgrave handbook of critical menstruation studies*, 2020, pp. 143–62.

P 255   The evidence backs this up: girls with . . .: M Larki et al., 'The relationship between menstrual patterns and menstrual attitude dimensions among women of reproductive age', *Sultan Qaboos University medical journal*, vol. 22, no. 2, 2022.

Index

fear of 12–14
medications and self-care
during 149–50
period management tool kit
279
period pain management,
non-pharmacological
279–80
period pain management,
supplements 280
remedies for period 149–54
song 252–3
yoga and meditation for 264–5
see also menstrual cycle,
retrograde menstruation
peripheral nervous system 111,
113
Perry, Bruce 195
polycystic ovarian syndrome
(PCOS) 51, 130, 158
polyvagal theory 112–13, 118,
120
Ponstan (mefenamic acid) 46,
150
Porges, Dr Stephen 112
post-traumatic stress disorder
(PTSD) 130, 132–3, 187,
194–5, 216
complex PTSD 133, 195
power, taking back 250–4
practitioners, guide to finding
282–7
probiotics 157
progesterone 5
progestin-only pills 52–4
possible side effects 53–4
risks of 53

prostaglandins 6–8, 17, 47, 93,
149, 159, 168, 212, 280
protective behaviours,
minimising 233–4
Provera (medroxyprogesterone
acetate) 52–3
PTSD *see* post-traumatic stress
disorder (PTSD)

R
resistance to change 81–2
retrograde menstruation 22–3,
32–5
Robins, Elissa 117, 174–5
Ryeqo 58

S
Sachs, Nicole 187
safety
how to return to your window
of tolerance 185–190
journaling on feelings of
182–3
resources for coming back to
290–1
returning to a state of 110,
118, 120–1, 169, 171–2,
177–8, 183–4, 191, 197,
202–3, 215, 217, 224,
237, 242, 245–7, 270
returning to safety exercise 190
tool kit to bring you back to
276–81
see also autonomic nervous
system, parasympathetic
state, ventral vagal state
Sampson, John 23